The Art and Science of Patient Education for Health Literacy

The Art and Science of Patient Education for Health Literacy

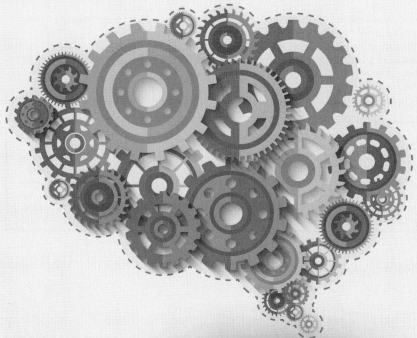

MELISSA N. STEWART, DNP, RN, CPE
Associate Professor and Award-Winning Health Literacy/Care
Transitions Consultant
Baton Rouge, Louisiana

ELSEVIER

Elsevier
3251 Riverport Lane
St. Louis, Missouri 63043

THE ART AND SCIENCE OF PATIENT EDUCATION FOR
HEALTH LITERACY, FIRST EDITION   ISBN: 978-0-323-60908-1

Notices

Practitioners and researchers must always rely on their own experience and knowledge in
evaluating and using any information, methods, compounds or experiments described herein.
Because of rapid advances in the medical sciences, in particular, independent verification of
diagnoses and drug dosages should be made. To the fullest extent of the law, no responsibility
is assumed by Elsevier, authors, editors or contributors for any injury and/or damage to
persons or property as a matter of products liability, negligence or otherwise, or from any use
or operation of any methods, products, instructions, or ideas contained in the material herein.

Library of Congress Control Number: 2019952853

Executive Content Strategist: Lee Henderson
Senior Content Development Manager: Luke Held
Senior Content Development Specialist: Jennifer Wade
Publishing Services Manager: Deepthi Unni
Project Manager: Radjan Lourde Selvanadin
Design Direction: Brian Salisbury

Working together
to grow libraries in
developing countries

www.elsevier.com • www.bookaid.org

Printed in the United States of America
Last digit is the print number: 9 8 7 6 5 4 3 2 1

Dawn Morris, PhD, MSN, BSN, RN, Instructor
Nursing Department
Louisiana State University
Eunice, Louisiana

Traci L. Alberti, PhD, FNP-BC
Assistant Professor,
  School of Health Sciences
Merrimack College
North Andover, Massachusetts

Sara L. Clutter, PhD, RN
Professor,
  Nursing Department
Waynesburg University
Waynesburg, Pennsylvania

Tanya Marie Cohn, PhD, M.Ed., RN
Nurse Scientist,
  Nursing and Health Sciences
  Research Department
Baptist Health South Florida
Miami, Florida;
Adjunct Faculty, College of Nursing
Simmons College
Boston, Massachusetts

Shawna Hughey, DNP, MSN, BSN, RN
Assistant Professor,
  Nursing Department
University of Arkansas at Pine Bluff
Pine Bluff, Arkansas

Nancy S. Morris, PhD, ANP-BC
Associate Professor, Adult Nurse
  Practitioner
Graduate School of Nursing
University of Massachusetts Medical
  School
Worcester, Massachusetts

Mariea Snell, DNP, MSN, FNP-C
Coordinator of Doctor of Nursing
  Practice Program, Assistant
  Professor of Nursing
Catherine McAuley School of
  Nursing, Myrtle E. and
  Earl E. Walker College of Health
  Professions
Maryville University
St. Louis, Missouri

CONTENTS

It was the best of times, it was the worst of times, it was the age of wisdom, it was the age of foolishness, it was the epoch of belief, it was the epoch of incredulity, it was the season of Light, it was the season of Darkness, it was the spring of hope, it was the winter of despair, we had everything before us, we had nothing before us....

CHARLES DICKENS
A Tale of Two Cities

MEDAGOGY

The Medagogy conceptual framework has been a work of the heart, a decade in the making. Before health literacy was a common term, my curiosity as a healthcare provider had already started questioning why patients were constantly returning to access points of care—as if they were in a frequent flyer rewards program.

The revolving door associated with recidivism continued as I pursued higher educational opportunities. In my graduate studies, I was exposed to learning and teaching theory that piqued my interest in patient teaching and the learning process. In my Master's degree studies, the PITS model served as the focus of my thesis. Simplicity of the model, coupled with the practicality of its use, stimulated appeals from colleagues for continued development and work in health literacy and patient education.

CARE TRANSITIONS SUCCESS

Although new to many, the Medagogy model is not new to healthcare. The Medagogy model has played an integral role in the success of the nationally recognized Centers for Medicaid and Medicare Systems (CMS) Care Transitions pilot. From coach to physician, all healthcare providers in the award-winning pilot were trained in the Medagogy model. The ease of application and implementation within a practice setting has made Medagogy the perfect fit for Care Transitions. Since the success of the pilot, the Medagogy model has been cited as the process that every healthcare provider should know and be held to for patient education.

This book is written for healthcare providers and is designed to walk the reader through empirically proven theoretical educational, psychological, and behavioral theories and the neurocognitive science of learning, which serve as the foundational support for the Medagogy structure. As the reader progresses through the book, fundamental parts of the Medagogy model will be introduced individually. The culmination of this journey is met when all the parts are presented together in a global overview of the Medagogy model, followed by the Understanding Personal Perspective (UPP) tool.

THE CENTER OF IT ALL: THE PATIENT

The Medagogy model serves to bridge the information gap between patients and healthcare providers. Integral parts of the Medagogy model, the health informational seasons, the patient education hierarchy, the PITS model, and the UPP tool serve to aid healthcare providers, individually and jointly, in their patient educational efforts. The model also serves to ensure that each patient is provided with the foundational information needed to make informed healthcare decisions.

Medagogy is built on empirically proven, age-old teaching, learning, psychological, and behavioral principles and theories. Replication of academic tools such as teaching plans, homework, and a report card system offer socially acceptable and familiar instruments known to aid in knowledge progression. The interdisciplinary synergism of information disbursement to patients as they progress through the healthcare continuum presents the opportunity for shared knowledge to occur in the patient-provider relationship.

Technology and advances in genetics have offered healthcare a glimpse into what could be the best of times in our industry. Every day, people's lives are being saved through the miracle of modern medicine. Unfortunately, a closer look reveals that healthcare also is facing the worst of times. Life is expensive, and healthy living is even more costly. The lives being saved and the knowledge being used to save them are leaving a strong fiscal imprint on our economy that reaches into all households.

Preventable errors and fragmented care are challenging our healthcare delivery system as we have transitioned into a new era, where quality and outcomes determine provider reimbursement. This new day in healthcare offers the promise of change. Alterations will occur in the dynamics among all players involved, from provider to patient.

This new edition includes the WHY patient self-activation tool, which will allow patients to gather the information they need to make informed decisions. The WHY activation tool assists the patient in gathering vital information that the PITS model covers. The WHY tool provides another process for patients' empowerment as they move along on their health journey.

STRENGTHENING THE PATIENT-PROVIDER BOND

Providers need to seek out strong relationships with the consumers of their services, both patients and other healthcare professionals. Nonchalant passive patients may prove to be a liability in our new healthcare paradigm because lack of engagement of the patient in the care relationship can result in less than optimal outcomes, which can equate to less reimbursement. Never has a strong relationship between provider and patient been needed as much as it is now.

Patients, along with their healthcare providers, must have a solid understanding of their health and how, as patients, they can influence their health status through behavior. Patients must be exposed to vital information that is used to drive the healthcare providers' diagnosis and treatment suggestions. Exposure to this data may be comforting, and understanding this information is empowering.

Truly informed decisions can occur only when complete transparency is present. One cannot make good decisions if the material is not understood. Lack of knowledge, on the part of the patient or provider, opens the door to error. Decisions made using incomplete knowledge are not informed decisions. With clarity of understanding, patients can apply value to their options and truly weigh their decisions based on their own quality of life definition and personal health goals.

Much like the aforementioned Dickens classic, healthcare is undergoing a revolution. Present transitions in healthcare are moving toward a true patient-centered delivery system. Medagogy focuses on meeting patients where they are in their health, in their knowledge, and in their goals. Health sustainability is contingent on responsible self-care. Patient education is the key to success in healthcare because it is the enabling factor that allows patients to assume their rightful position of control in their healthcare treatment.

For more information about Medagogy, please visit www.organizationof-patienteducators.com.

Shifting the Focus to the Patient

CHAPTER 1

The Problem of Health Literacy

Health is an elusive concept in which there is no one universal definition. Health has been defined as a state of well-being, optimal physical conditioning, and desired shape and strength. Much like beauty, health is in the eye of the beholder, meaning personal interpretation ultimately impacts individual meaning. Historically, the healthcare system has assumed a role of authority and expertise in the acquisition of health. Through knowledge, expertise, and influence, healthcare providers attempt to assist people in their quest for health often without knowing what the consumer of their service, the patient, is actually seeking when they access the healthcare setting.

For years, healthcare providers have talked of partnering with the consumers of their services, their patients. Partnering brings to the relationship a sense of equality and shared control. Unfortunately, the variety of individual knowledge and perspectives has served as barriers to the partnership. The lack of shared understanding has impeded the provider and the patient's ability to merge their health perceptions into a unified effort to achieve the "health" that the patient is seeking.

Never has the need for a provider-patient partnership been greater than right now. As healthcare moves from a reactive health-delivery model, where treatment begins when a health insult occurs, toward a proactive delivery model, where the prevention of health insults and disease onset is the focus, change must occur in our present form of healthcare delivery. To achieve optimal outcomes with this shift in healthcare delivery, the provider and patient must be in sync with their healthcare goals and agreed-upon treatments. Lack of understanding on either part, provider or patient, can hinder progress toward desired health results. A foundation of shared understanding can be achieved by improving patient education through established definitions and structures. Ideal patient education would be delivered as the patient accesses healthcare. The information would be delivered using a common pathway that can be replicated and reinforced at every access point by the healthcare provider team. Each provider would build on and reinforce his or her previous patient-education efforts using repetition, the oldest law of learning. Through knowledge building and reinforcement, patients become empowered and can truly partner with their providers as they are able to make informed decisions. For preventive medicine and provider-patient partnerships to occur, progression of patient knowledge through patient education must become a focus of the healthcare industry.

Patient health knowledge is the subject of interest in this book. It will focus on the information-exchange process that occurs in the patient-provider relationship in the healthcare system. Throughout the chapters, the process of patient education according to the *medagogy* model will be reviewed. The medagogy model works to identify information flow throughout the process of patient education. The concepts and relationships of medagogy serve as the core of a training program for patient educators—the Certified Patient Educator (CPE) program.

Today, healthcare is a focus of national concern. Rudimentary problems such as inappropriate access with lack of fair and prudent resource utilization plague our present healthcare delivery model ("Access," 2005; Beyer, 2009; Bodenheimer and Fernandez, 2005; Evans, 2004; Ginsburg, 2004; Hanks, 1994; Lambrew, 2004; McLaughlin, 2008; Twanmoh and Cunningham, 2006; White, 1999). Proposed solutions to meeting the growing health needs of the nation and the world include greater access to providers, improved insurance coverage, and improved preventive services (Bailey, 1995; Esposito et al., 2006; Lancaster, et al., 2009; Thompson, et al., 2009). Although these proposed solutions can assist in addressing present healthcare concerns, movement toward active patient involvement can help relieve the present dependency of patients on healthcare services that has exhausted our healthcare system (Prilleltensky, 2005). The public's dependency on the healthcare system has been linked to poor health literacy. For the healthcare delivery system to move toward the new proactive delivery approach, massive systemic change must occur (Karpf et al., 2009; Lofgen et al., 2006).

Initially, healthcare providers need to look beyond the boundaries of their practice setting and past the present moment in time and into the future of healthcare for each patient they see. Although the patient may present with an acute condition, preventive healthcare will require the healthcare provider to make a time-oriented change in treatment focus to include present care and prospective health needs. Health-promotion and disease prevention success lie in early intervention (Breslow, 1999; Maibach et al., 2006). Point-of-service treatment will not be limited to the patient's past and present health as has been historically seen in healthcare; it must include proactive steps for patients' future health concerns. An individual patient's presenting health status, lifestyle, and family history are a few pieces of data that can help a provider to identify future health risks. Providers will need to address and prepare the patient for future health conditions that prospectively may threaten the patient's future health. Through education, providers can prepare patients for present and prospective health issues along with possible challenges that may be encountered in the future.

Flu-Like Symptoms Are an Opportunity to Educate a 45-year Old About Other Serious Health Risks

John, the town's chief of police, is a 45-year-old African-American male presenting with a history of high blood pressure, a family history of maternal and paternal heart disease, and a pack-a-day cigarette habit, is in the clinic for a chief complaint of flu-like symptoms. Although flu-like symptoms are the reason that the patient accessed the system and are his immediate treatment needs, the profile from his history and his lifestyle habits provide an opportunity to establish proactive interventions for the identified risks that may lead to future health problems. If the risks progress into actual diseases, the patient may lose more than his optimal health status. The transition from risk to actual health problems can rob the patient of quality of life, independence, financial security, and even life itself. The providers' glimpse into the potential future for this patient's health behaviors warrants action. The treatment of the acute state flu-like symptoms is the first priority because that is the patient's main concern. However, investing in the patient's future health by empowering him with information may save his life.

Expert Support for Action

Cardiovascular disease research consistently references stabilizing acute conditions before initiating any prevention (O'Keefe et al., 2009; Raczynski and DiClemente, 1999).

Falvo (2004) asserts that patient education focused on prevention is more effective if the patient's perceived needs and immediate concerns are addressed first.

Treatment

John is treated for his flu-like symptoms. After internist Dr. Flowers teaches John what is causing his present symptoms, signs that his condition may be worsening, action to take if symptoms worsen, schedules follow-up, and explains how to carry out his ordered treatment plan, he tells John that his history and lifestyle put him at risk for cardiac disease and long-term complications. Dr. Flowers then establishes with John the intent to focus on prospective cardiac issues on his next visit. On John's follow-up visit, his assessment reveals that John's initial health issue is resolved, so Dr. Flowers begins to expose him to information regarding his cardiac risk.

Ultimately, the provider of healthcare services will need to take past and present information from the patient's health history, clinical and laboratory findings, observed signs, and the patient's symptoms to render an expert opinion for present and future health needs.

Patients need to be as independent as possible in their healthcare, although there may be times that the patient may regress to a more dependent state, as in the case of a severe acute myocardial infarction (AMI) (Falvo, 2004). In the treatment of a severe AMI, the patient is totally dependent on the health-care provider; the only thing a patient can do in this case is follow directions and answer questions. Once the AMI is stabilized and the situation is under control, then the patient is more likely to be able to assume some self-care. Simple activities of daily living, such as brushing teeth and combing hair, are tasks that the patient may be able to resume.

When the patient is no longer in a critical health situation, the patient and the provider should partner to maximize the opportunity for improved health status. Healthcare providers need to look beyond the physical assessment, so the provider can tailor treatment to meet the patient's individual health needs (Falvo, 2004; Redman, 2004). Values, goals, priorities, and idiosyncrasies that are specific to that individual will provide direction for health resolution, disease prevention, health-promotion, and health maintenance. To meet the provider's informational needs, the patient will need to educate the provider about his or her condition, lifestyle, and personal habits that could impact his or her health status. The patient's understanding of self will serve to help guide the provider as the patient participates in the planning of his or her individual care. Likewise, the provider, who serves as the healthcare expert in the patient-provider relationship, will need to educate the patient on the functions of his or her body, how disease impacts its functions, and how suggested treatment options can help address the patient's health. Together, the two experts will forge a treatment plan oriented to the patient's life and the provider's understanding of applicable patient ability and resources.

The patient, as the expert of self, bears responsibility in the patient-provider relationship to educate the provider on himself or herself and personal life values and/or situations; the provider is obligated to give the patient a full rationale for the suggested treatment plan—the why behind the actions the patient will need to carry out. Possessing an understanding of why something should be done affords the patient the opportunity to prioritize this health information into his or her world. Redman (2004) recognizes the healthcare professional as the gatekeeper of healthcare knowledge. A patient's lack of exposure to healthcare professional rationale or knowledge limits the patient's power in his or her healthcare. Patient education empowers patients, so they are able to influence the direction and course of their personal healthcare, thereby increasing their health autonomy. Conversely, lack of exposure to provider rationale or knowledge can limit the patient's power in his or her healthcare.

Through active expert exchange of information in the patient-provider relationship, a common ground of understanding can be achieved. This common understanding is called shared knowledge. The healthcare system is the milieu for patient-care transitioning. The healthcare system must master the exchange of patient and treatment information between healthcare providers, entities, and systems. The informational hand-off between providers should include historical and present physical health status, treatment, and the progression of patient knowledge. Exchange of patient knowledge can offer a foundation upon which to build new information. Being aware of where the patient is in receiving information and understanding about his or her health allows providers who follow to build on the efforts of previous human resources focused on educating the patient before the present encounter. It is well documented in the literature that healthcare providers at various points of care either over- or underestimate patients' understanding of their health and their desire for information (Keulers et al., 2008; Schwartzberg, 2002).

In the ideal progression of the patient health-knowledge delivery model, provider understanding of previous educational efforts by the patient would allow new teaching efforts to refresh and expand on the prior work of other providers. Each provider would build on the patient's knowledge, allowing the patient to move toward higher levels of comprehension and independence regarding his or her health and self-care. The system supports the provider's and the patient's knowledge progression as they move toward a common domain of shared knowledge. Figure 1.1 displays the shared knowledge domain necessary for the provider and the patient to create a healthcare plan in a partnership.

Patient education is a basic yet vital element of healthcare that must be addressed to ensure success in healthcare (Smith et al., 2009). In the challenge of creating a new, divergent healthcare delivery system, patient education can facilitate our passage into a new paradigm of healthcare—a paradigm where healthcare is constructed around a provider-patient relationship and where health goals and treatment choices are the products of a mutually shared and gained understanding (Prilleltensky, 2005). *Shared knowledge* is defined as

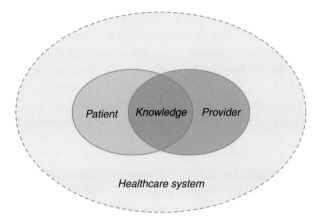

Fig. 1.1   Shared knowledge domains. The domains of knowledge for patient, provider, and healthcare system are displayed. Provider and patient are working within the healthcare system. The intersection of the provider, the patient, and the healthcare system depicts the common knowledge shared by all three domains.

general information universally understood by all parties. It is identified in the illustration of Figure 1.1 as portions of individual circle representations that intersect, sharing a common space that represents the knowledge that is shared by all three parties: the patient, the provider, and the healthcare system. The knowledge shared between the patient, provider, and healthcare system serves as a foundation upon which new knowledge can be constructed. Shared knowledge is also a connection between parties, which can be used to gain more pertinent knowledge about one another.

In the healthcare system, the shared domain of knowledge between experts—the provider and the patient—allows for assigned control and power to both parties in the partnership. Only the patient knows what he or she truly wants to gain in his or her healthcare; therefore, people need to maintain the right to manage their health by maintaining control of their healthcare (Cagle and Kovacs, 2009). Patient education is a conduit to help patients assume their rightful collaborative role in the patient-provider relationship. Patient education has moved from its narrow medical illness-related origin of patient teaching to a broader paradigm of personal empowerment and participation, inclusive of health-promotion, self-care, and disease prevention (Cagle and Kovacs, 2009; Roter et al., 2001).

Health literacy is a term that is used to communicate a level of proficiency with a skill associated with healthcare and/or health maintenance. Presently, the term *health literacy* represents the level of competency in health maintenance that a patient possesses. The receiver of health services, the patient, is the focus of health literacy in today's healthcare setting. Health literacy does not occur in a vacuum, but instead, health literacy problems are exacerbated as a patient cycles through the healthcare system desperately seeking a solution to his or her defined health needs. The maze of broken communication and inconsistency among providers in our reactive delivery system perpetuates confusion and compounds the unrealistic expectations placed on patients. True success in healthcare today requires clear communication from both parties in the provider-patient partnership.

Identifying which skills the patient lacks is only one aspect of addressing the patient's health literacy. The provider's knowledge deficit of the patient's interpretation of health needs, patient values, and how behavioral changes fit into the patient's definition of quality of life are other patient issues that must be addressed. To better appreciate the need for an informed patient, the problem of health literacy needs to be examined in detail.

Health Literacy Today

Health literacy is defined by the US Department of Health and Human Services, the National Library of Medicine, the Center for Health Care Strategies, and the Institute of Medicine (IOM) has the aptitude to gain, interpret, and use basic health information and understand what assistance is needed to make appropriate healthcare decisions (Centers for Disease Control, 2007; Center for Health Strategies, Inc., 2005; Mancuso, 2008; US Department of Health and Human Services, 2008). The World Health Organization (WHO) includes patient motivation (Kickbusch, 2001) in health literacy, whereas the American Medical Association (AMA) adds the ability to measure and use numeracy to their definition (Greenburg, 2001; Mancuso, 2008). Nutbeam (2000) inserts personal life context into his health literacy definition, which adds the individual situation and priorities to the patient's health status. This paragraph shows that health literacy has various meanings and definitions with no common construct, making it a challenge to measure and fully study (Baker, 2006). Healthy People 2010, a program launched by the US Department of Health and Human Services includes goals to improve the health literacy crisis (Centers for Disease Control, 2007). Healthy People 2020 retains the health literacy objectives of Healthy People 2010 and added them under the heading of health communication/health information technology initiatives (Secretary's Advisory Committee on National Health Promotion and Disease Prevention, 2009).

The following definition takes into account the skills needed from all the parties involved in healthcare. Health literacy is the patient's level of health understanding, inclusive of personal values and priorities that then frames health decisions and results in health action through behavioral change determined from individual interpretation. The provider and the patient both use their values and knowledge to make healthcare decisions. Actions resulting from decisions are determined from personal meaning. Health choices can impact quality of life. Behavioral change driven by health choices may range from extreme to no action. For whatever action is chosen, the choice lies with the beholder because quality of life is individually defined. If either party does not view the requested action as a priority, then a struggle between provider and patient goals may ensue. Mutual health goals established through the acceptance of each party's values and choices can deliver achievable health outcomes. A lack of health literacy is not a deficit on the patient's part, instead it is a deficit resulting from both the patient and provider. Rudd (2015) acknowledges that health literacy outcomes are representative of the literacy skills and communication skills of both patients and providers.

To benefit from everything healthcare has to offer, health literacy skills are vital for the patient (Boswell et al., 2004; Tkacz et al., 2008). We are all affected by health literacy because our health is a part of everyday life. According to the CDC (2016), even people who read well and are comfortable with numbers may face health literacy issues because of the following:

- Being unfamiliar with medical terms, technical information, and/or how their body works.
- Inability to interpret statistics and evaluate risks and benefits that affect their health and safety.
- Being scared and confused because they have been diagnosed with a serious illness.
- Having health conditions that require complicated self-care.

History of Health Literacy

Health literacy has been a catchphrase since it was first uttered in 1974 (Simonds, 1978), and the lack of health literacy is a colossal problem in healthcare in the United States and around the world (Carter and Wallace, 2007; Betz et al., 2008). In the 1990s, the field of health literacy became a trendy focus for research in response to society's sobering new awareness of the strong association between health and education (White, 2008). In 1998, seven statements were incorporated into the Patient's Bill of Rights as introduced by the American Hospital Association (AHA), which addressed information patients receive, and acknowledged a patient's right to know about their health status, care options, and requirements for care (US Department of Health and Human Services, 1999). Health literacy expert Osborne (2005) acknowledges the importance of health literacy by heightening awareness that life-threatening mistakes happen when patients cannot read or comprehend health information. Even well-educated people have difficulty understanding medical jargon, medical forms, and prescription information (Burnham and Peterson, 2005; Committee on Health Literacy, 2004). Barrett and Puryear (2006) state that all patients, from the well educated to those with limited literacy skills, are vulnerable to misunderstanding, incomprehension, and not being able to act on healthcare provider directions. Clear patient-oriented provider communication offers an opportunity to decrease this lack of understanding and confusion in the patient population (Barrett and Puryear, 2006; Sudore and Schillinger, 2009).

Health Literacy Internationally

Health illiteracy is not endemic to the United States. On the contrary, it is a health crisis that crosses borders throughout the world. Switzerland, Australia, New Zealand, and other countries are also struggling with the challenge of health literacy (Stableford and Mettger, 2007). Canadian and European patients may have easier access to healthcare through their nationalized healthcare systems, but these regions also deal with health illiteracy as their healthcare consumers struggle to read, understand, and use information essential to preventing, treating, and properly managing complex health conditions. The WHO and the European Commission reports highlight that effective communication is critical to public understanding of health information (Stableford and Mettger, 2007). The American Institute of Medicine, Agency for Healthcare Research and Quality (AHRQ), and the Health Association Libraries Section, a section of the Medical Library Association, all have produced reports that stress the same need as the reports of the WHO and the European Commission—a need for clear, congruent, legitimate information (Stableford and Mettger, 2007) that is relevant and culturally competent.

The Canadian Public Health Association (CPHA) claims that low health literacy is a serious and costly problem that will become worse as the Canadian population ages and the incidence of chronic disease proliferates (Fitzpatrick, 2008). The CPHA proposes that improving health literacy will lead to decreased healthcare costs and improved outcomes. Enhanced communication can improve health literacy and can ultimately reduce a nation's overall healthcare burden by decreasing dependency on healthcare by empowering people with health skills (Furnee et al., 2008; Monachos, 2007).

The IOM and the AHRQ, two major agencies in the US healthcare system, both issued health literacy reports in 2004 that placed the topic of health literacy at the forefront of the nation's health agenda (Stableford and Mettger, 2007). The WHO's 6th annual global conference acknowledged that health-promoting strategies provide equal learning opportunities for all people to achieve basic health literacy and are an essential duty for all levels of government (Stableford and Mettger, 2007). The WHO report notes that clear, uninhibited communication is a critical component of effective promotion of health (Stableford and Mettger, 2007). Effective health provider communication strategies are essential to mobilize people toward healthy options and increase the likelihood of choices that could produce healthy behaviors (Stableford and Mettger, 2007).

Prevalence of Health Literacy

Unlike a broken arm, an abnormal blood pressure, or even elevated blood glucose, there are no physical signs or symptoms to alert a healthcare provider to a silent, costly, crippling, even deadly health problem: a lack of health literacy. There is no age, no race, no gender, no face, and there is little to no social differentiation between a person who is health literate and one who has poor health literacy. Although found in all segments of society, those persons born and raised in the United States represent the majority of the population with poor health literacy (Weiss, 2009). In the United States, poor health literacy is characterized as the "silent epidemic" of public health (Marcus, 2006). The percentage of people with insufficient health-literacy skills increased from 40% of the US adult population in 1992 to greater than 50% in 2004, or approximately 90 million people (Maniaci et al., 2008). The 2003 National Healthcare Disparities Report from the National Assessment of Adult Health Literacy found that 12% of Americans have proficient health-literacy skills, 53% have intermediate skills, and 36% have basic to low health literacy skills (AHRQ, 2006; Health literacy in the United States, 2008). Maniaci et al. (2008) state that advances in healthcare technology and complications of healthcare delivery have made it increasingly difficult to assess a patient's ability to understand complex medical information.

Education Impact on Health Literacy in the United States

Evidence supports a positive relationship between education and health (Furnee et al., 2008). According to the US Department of Labor, 47% of the adult population of the United States has poor literacy, and 10% to 14% of adults in the workforce have a learning disability. One out of every five patients is functionally illiterate (Kirsch et al., 2002). A study of 445 adult female subjects with fourth-grade literacy skills found that 39% did not understand why women get mammograms (Davis et al., 1998). A study of 3260 elderly subjects found a relationship between educational attainment and health status (Howard et al., 2006).

Literacy level is not always reflective of educational level, but is strongly associated with employment, community membership, and health status (Health Canada, 1999). A 2002 study that reviewed claims for a Medicare-managed care company for 2 years found that enrollees who had low literacy had a 52% higher risk of hospital admission (Baker et al., 2002). Of chronically ill American adults, 75% possess low literacy skills (Cutilli and Bennett, 2009; Prasauskas and Spoo, 2006).

Most health education is written at a high school level, whereas the average Medicaid recipient reads at a fifth-grade level (US Department of Labor, 2001). The average Medicare recipient reads at a sixth-grade level (GAO, 2006). To add to the complexity, healthcare has its own language, which is unfamiliar to most people. Patient education products often burden the reader with confusing complex medical verbiage.(Schwartzenburg et al., 2005). A 1997 study discovered that even college-educated individuals have difficulty interpreting and using medical information (Schwartz et al., 1997).

It is not uncommon for patients to hide their incomprehension and literacy limitations because of shame or embarrassment (Kripalani and Weiss, 2006). Unfortunately, most healthcare professionals are not trained to help patients deal with their feelings of shame related to literacy, nor are they trained on how to communicate with a patient struggling with health-literacy issues (Schwartzenberg et al., 2007). It is common for patients to not admit that they do not understand what the provider is saying or directing them to do. Unfortunately, these patients admit that they feel inept and incapable of asking their healthcare provider questions or requesting clarification (Leydon et al., 2000; McKenzie, 2000).

Ethnic and Elder Disparity

Poor health literacy has been found to be more common in ethnic minorities, the impoverished, and the elderly (Committee on Understanding and Eliminating Racial and Ethnic Disparities in Health Care, 2003; Schillinger et al., 2002). One study found that 42% of 202 African Americans surveyed acknowledged inadequate health literacy (Parikh et al., 1996). The growth in poor health literacy skills is rapidly outpacing advances in healthcare technology; therefore, to meet the patient's basic need to understand, healthcare providers must concentrate their efforts on addressing the problem of health literacy through scientific exploration of potential solutions (Greenburg, 2001; Raynor, 2008; Sorrell, 2006). Low health literacy presents challenges to medication identification (Kripalani et al., 2006) and to medication self-management (Davis and Wolf, 2006; Kripalani et al., 2006; Wolf et al., 2007). A study of 85 subjects using discussion group participants with low literacy found medication labels confusing and difficult to understand (Webb et al., 2008). Another study found that by addressing medication misunderstandings, clinicians created a foundation on which to build new knowledge so that patients can be more self-sufficient in their care (Spiers et al., 2004).

The Financial Impact of Health Literacy

Health spending in the United States is expected to top the overall national market increase by 3% per year, resulting in growth from 13% of gross domestic product (GDP) in 2009 to 17% in 2010 (Gross Domestic Report: Third Quarter 2009, 2009; National Health Expenditure Data, 2010). Low health literacy inflicts a heavy financial impact on healthcare cost. A report entitled, *Health Literacy: A Prescription to End Confusion*, released by the Institute of Medicine, estimated that the health literacy problem generates an annual cost of $73 billion dollars (Committee on Health Literacy, 2004). In 2007, the estimated annual price tag of low health literacy increased to approximately $106 to $236 billion (Vernon et al., 2007). These funds are spent because patients do not understand the communications and expectations of their healthcare providers (Roberts, 2004). Likewise, providers do not know what the patient does not know, nor does the provider know how the patient may feel about prescribed actions to be performed for a successful treatment plan.

The costs and utilization of healthcare services tracked through claims files by the participants revealed that enrollees with inadequate health-literacy skills incurred higher medical costs than those with adequate health-literacy skills (Howard et al., 2005). The Short Test of Functional Health Literacy was used to measure 3260 participants' health literacy, revealing that 800 subjects had inadequate health-literacy skills, 366 subjects had marginal health-literacy skills, and 2094 subjects had adequate health-literacy skills. The cost and utilization of healthcare services were then tracked through the participants' claim files. The data revealed that subjects with inadequate health-literacy skills incurred higher medical costs when compared with enrollees with adequate health-literacy skills (Howard et al., 2005). Individuals with limited health-literacy skills have difficulty understanding their medication labels, suffer increased risks of hospitalization related to misunderstandings about health self-care, and use fewer preventive services (Harper, 2007).

People with poor health literacy or diminished health understanding are directly impacted because they experience less than optimal health outcomes (Schwartzberg, 2002). The lack of understanding of how to take medicine correctly or read food labels to maintain dietary restrictions are two examples of common health-literacy errors. Everyone is affected by the financial impact caused by inappropriate use and access of the healthcare system, increased length of stay (Weiss et al., 1994), extra healthcare provider visits (Harper, 2007), and recidivism (Baker et al., 2002; Weiss et al., 1994).

Although copious data help to identify the problem and its ravenous consumption of healthcare resources, low health literacy remains a major issue. A lack of patient understanding leads to return visits, recidivism, increased financial burden, and less than optimal health outcomes (Harper, 2007). Healthcare reform offers an opportunity for patient education to become a central priority in healthcare. Improving health literacy can decrease a nation's overall healthcare costs (Furnee et al., 2008; Monachos, 2007).

As healthcare costs continue to surge, there is an underlying acknowledgment that consumers must become active participants in their own healthcare. Healthcare reform continues to be a monumental paradigm shift that aims to transition our nation's healthcare from a reactive delivery system to a patient-centered, proactive, preventive, predictive model. To achieve a healthcare environment where consumers and providers both participate in treatment decision making, patients must have a better understanding of their health status, and providers must have a good understanding of the patient's perspective and self-efficacy to adhere to a treatment regimen (Boswell et al., 2004; Tkacz et al., 2008).

Recognizing the need for the provider to learn from the patient is a major challenge that may aid in resolving the issue of poor health literacy. It is crucial for the provider to learn from the patient, to understand the patient's perspective, and to act upon patient-communicated information. Personal information from the patient can assist the provider in the formulation of a truly individualized plan of care (Redman, 2004). Information shared between the patient and provider forms the foundation of understanding from which both parties draw healthcare conclusions. The provider develops treatment options from information received from the patient. The patient creates personal relevance from the information received from the provider.

There must be congruence and a sense of mutual trust between the two individuals for good communication to occur. Good communication can lead to better health outcomes with each interaction. Through knowledge empowerment, patient and provider can remove barriers and move toward commonly defined and accepted health goals.

Summary

- Much like beauty, health is in the eye of the beholder, meaning personal interpretation ultimately impacts individual meaning.
- Never has the need for a provider-patient partnership been more needed than now. As healthcare moves from a reactive delivery model to a proactive delivery model, the provider and patient must be in sync to achieve optimal health outcomes.
- Throughout the book, the process of patient education according to the medagogy model will be reviewed. The medagogy model works to identify information flow throughout the process of patient education.
- When the patient is no longer in a critical health situation, the patient and the provider should partner to maximize the opportunity for improved health status.
- Through active expert exchange of information in the patient-provider relationship, a common ground of understanding can be achieved. This common understanding is called shared knowledge.
- Well documented in the literature is the fact that healthcare providers at various points of care either over- or underestimate the patients' understanding of their health and their desire for information
- In the healthcare system, the shared domain of knowledge between experts—the provider and the patient—allocate assigned control and power to both parties in the partnership.
- *Health literacy* is the level of health understanding, inclusive of personal values and priorities that then frames health decisions and results in health action through behavioral change as determined by individual interpretation. The provider and patient both use their values and knowledge to make healthcare decisions.
- Clear patient-oriented provider communication offers an opportunity to decrease the lack of understanding and confusion in the patient population.

CHAPTER 2

The Patient's Perspective

Health literacy needs to move from being disease oriented to being patient oriented. In fact, the term *health literacy* should be exchanged for the term *patient literacy*. The focus should be on formulating information specific to that patient: educators must be sure to consider who, where, and how the patient is at this particular point in time or season of health. Each patient needs education, and it is crucial to plan and deliver the necessary information based on that person's physical and psychological situation at that moment in time.

Does New Mom Training in Diaper Changing?

Jamie is a new mother. Like all new mothers, Jamie needs to understand how to change a baby's diaper. Jamie, however, has experience changing babies' diapers. She works in the daycare by the hospital and lives next door to her sister who has three small children. By including Jamie's experience when evaluating her patient-education needs, we may help a healthcare team focus on knowledge needs that are more appropriate for her. Compared with other first-time mothers, Jamie does not require as much information regarding diaper changing.

EXPERT SUPPORT FOR ACTION

Patient education is a legal responsibility of every licensed healthcare provider (Kraut, 1981). The US Joint Commission on Accreditation of Healthcare Organizations requires accredited health institutions to identify and address each patient's health knowledge needs and encourages healthcare providers to partner with patients through information exchange and active patient participation in planning and execution of healthcare (The Joint Commission, 2007). The more that is known about the patient, the more the information can be personalized (Boothman, 2002). To have a constructive dialogue, a platform of shared knowledge is required between provider and patient (Makoul, 2003). Providers need to gain an understanding of the patient from the information each patient provides (Hahn, 2009; Weiner et al., 2005).

8-Year-Old W/Asthma

Surprisingly, skill does not always increase with age. For instance, Ashley, an 8-year-old girl with asthma, is quite proficient with the use of her inhaler. Ashley has suffered with asthma since the age of 5. Over the years, Ashley has not only mastered using her inhaler, but she also knows how to identify when her body is telling her she needs to use the inhaler. Ashley has become so comfortable with her inhaler skill that she helped her neighbor Joe, a 30-year-old man newly diagnosed with asthma when he could not figure out how to activate his inhaler.

EXPERT SUPPORT FOR ACTION

Through knowledge, a patient can cope with health and altered health states, which can improve health outcomes and enhance quality of life (Cooper et al., 2001). There is no age, no race, no sex, no face, and there is little to no social differentiation between a person who is health literate and one who is not (Stewart, 2012).

There is a need to transition patient education from a global, standardized, one-size-fits-all model to an individually focused effort tailored specifically for each person. Maniaci et al. (2008) affirm that adequate patient-centered communication is needed to improve patient understanding. Patients must have an adequate level of understanding of their medical circumstances to interact effectively with their healthcare providers and to actively participate in their healing process. Maniaci et al. (2008) assert that a patient's ability to understand his or her circumstances can impact independence, safety, cost of care, and overall health outcomes.

Health literacy is still evolving, and it is crucial to resolve the issue of patients not understanding their health status or their health-status provider recommendations, which result in patients' dependence on the healthcare system (Center for Disease Control, 2007; Center for Health Strategies, Inc., 2005; Mancuso, 2008; US Department of Health and Human Services, 2008). In an attempt to address health literacy, Edmunds (2005) proposes that all health material for the general population be written and communicated at fifth- to seventh-grade levels to improve the odds of patients understanding the content. Empirical literature substantiates the opposite position—that limited universal levels are not effective for all patients (Billek-Sawhney and Reicherter, 2005; Hoffman and McKenna, 2006; Kolm, and Jacobson, 2008; Kripalani et al., 2001).

Mayer advocates for providers to meet the individual patient at his or her level of need (Roberts, 2004), which would require healthcare educator training in the assessment skills of patients' learning needs and information delivery for healthcare providers. Because people have varying learning styles and different literacy levels, patient education needs to be designed to accommodate each individual's educational capabilities (Kurashige, 2008). Studies show that individualized instructions increase comprehension and memory more effectively than standardized instructions (Morrow et al, 2005; Robinson et al., 2008). Healthcare providers need to present information in a manner in which each patient can understand, recall, and use in his or her life and in making healthcare choices (Stableford and Mettger, 2007).

Empirical data identifying the seriousness of the health-literacy crisis have prompted an appeal for trained healthcare providers to effectively educate patients (Kripalani et al., 2008; Schillinger et al., 2003; Visser et al., 2001). Baker et al. (2002, p. 1283) assert that "it may be beneficial to think of limited health literacy analogously to physical disabilities: wheelchair-bound patients are not expected to climb stairs to access healthcare". Similar to the accommodations that are mandated for patients with disabilities, "health care information should be made available to all patients regardless of their reading ability" (Baker et al., 2002, p. 1283).

Providers of health services need to value the power, an educator can bring to patient knowledge. It is assumed that if a healthcare provider knows a patient's literacy level, he or she can make adjustments so the information the patient receives will match the patient's literacy level (Greenburg, 2001). A study of 182 diabetic patients and 63 physicians revealed that physicians did not feel they possessed the skills needed to adequately adapt information to each patient's educational needs (Seligman et al., 2005). Most healthcare providers do not know how to adjust information or engage in patient teaching using educational principles and theories. A metaanalysis reviewed multiple types of patient educational interventions and found that theoretical models and educational frameworks were absent (Cooper et al., 2001). Educational theory is necessary to guide patient teaching (Glanz et al., 2008). Personalized and theoretically grounded patient education is important to resolve the health literacy problem (Committee on Health Literacy, 2004).

Controversy exists regarding whether healthcare providers receive adequate training to be good patient educators (Chang and Kelly, 2007; Luker and Caress, 1988). Although healthcare providers may be a valuable source of information, more training may be needed to allow them to be truly effective in patient education (Luker and Caress, 1988).

Patient Education

Skillful patient education can empower patients with health knowledge and control (Falvo, 1994; Redman, 2006; Marcus, 2014). Healthcare providers often ad lib the educational segments of their services to patients and fail to assign appropriate importance to this responsibility. This is unfortunate because patients rely on the information they receive from their providers. Knowledge dispersed by providers often serves as the foundation on which patients gain the knowledge and information they need to independently manage their personal healthcare needs (Kripalani and Weiss, 2006; Makoul, 2003). Unlike many other skills applied in healthcare, there is no global definition for the skill of patient education (Makoul, 2003). The National League of Nursing (NLN), in their 1976 publication, *Patient Education*, defined *patient education* as the 'process of providing patients with the knowledge, skill, competence, or desirable qualities of behavior.' Phillips (1999) points out that patient teaching is the activity that is done to facilitate patient learning. Redman (2006) distinguishes patient education as a process of influence and planned learning. Redman further states that in the patient education experience, a combination of methods and techniques is used to influence patient knowledge and behavior (Redman, 2006). Patient education is also defined as "all educational activities, directed to patients, including aspects of therapeutic education, health education, and clinical health-promotion" (Deccache and Aujoulat, 2001, p. 8). According to Bastable (2006, p. 466), patient education is "the process of assisting consumers of health care to learn how to incorporate health-related behaviors into everyday life with the purposes of achieving the goal of optimal health."

For the purposes of this book, patient education is defined as the act of purposeful patient engagement in activities that can impact patients' knowledge through personal learning for future use, health autonomy, and long-term retention. Patient learning includes the individual, along with the personal processes of mental ingestion and absorption of planned and unplanned information.

Brief Reflections on Patient Education History

In the 18th and 19th centuries, verbal communication and observation were the main sources of information for patient diagnosis and treatment (Reiser, 1981). Through the years, technology has threatened the relationship between patient and provider, distancing the relationship, while stifling verbal exchange. The participation of nursing in the practice of patient education is noted in the literature as far back as 1900 in the *American Journal of Nursing* (1[1]), in an article entitled "Visiting nursing" by Eliza J. Moore. However, according to Falvo (1994), actual documentation within patient charts of nurses providing patient education only dates back to the early 1950s.

In the 1960s, the civil rights movement helped thrust social equality and empowerment into all areas of society, including healthcare (Rosen, 1977). During this period, the American Medical Association (AMA) established an ethical commitment to patient education. In the 1970s, the focus shifted to increasing awareness of patient education and patient rights, especially with the 1971 publication of *The Need for Patient Education* by the US Department of Health, Education, and Welfare (Falvo, 1994). In 1973, the American Hospital Association (AHA) developed *The Patient's Bill of Rights* (American Hospital Association, 1973). Also in 1973, the American Nurses Association (ANA) published *ANA's Standards of Nursing Practice*, which identified nurses' responsibilities in patient education (American Nurses Association, 1973). The patient's bill of rights became regarded as an ethical guide to the delivery of healthcare through honoring patients' rights to information, involvement, and choice (NLN, 1976).

In 1975, the ANA published *The Professional Nurse and Health Education*, which delineated patient education as a responsibility of the registered nurse from illness to health maintenance (ANA, 2004; Falvo, 1994). The 1975, ANA publications also indicated accountability on the part of the nurse, the patient, and family for delivery of relevant appropriate information throughout the healthcare process (American Nurses Association, 1975). In 1980, the AMA sanctioned a new version of the *Principles of Medical Ethics*, calling for physicians to make healthcare information available for patients. The Patient Self-Determination Act was enacted in December 1991. This act enabled patients to make choices about end-of-life issues, such as life support and other life-sustaining interventions, through advanced directives (Markus, 1997). In March 1998, the Patient's Bill of Rights became law (US Department of Health and Human Services, 1999). Since then, all licensed healthcare providers are required to educate patients as outlined in the seven statements in the patient's bill of rights.

The focus of health literacy should deal with information that the patient receives, while acknowledging the patient's right to know about personal health problems, health status, treatments, alternative care options, and continuing care requirements (US Department of Health and Human Services, 1999). Figure 2.1 displays a timeline in health-literacy education.

Although patient education has been part of the standards of The Joint Commission (TJC) since 1976 (Joint Commission on Accreditation of Healthcare Organizations, 1976), in March 2002, the Centers for Medicare and Medicaid, in partnership with TJC, launched a national public campaign called "Speak Up" (TJC, 2010). The campaign was designed as a patient safety initiative to help prevent medical errors and healthcare mistakes by

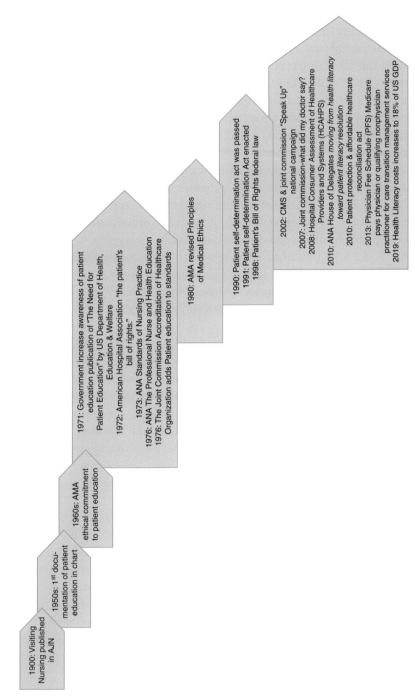

Fig. 2.1 Patient education timeline provides a historical review of events that are significant to patient education. (Falvo, 2004; Moore, 1900; Redman, 2004).

urging the lay population to get involved in their healthcare by asking questions and actively participating in their healthcare planning (TJC, 2010).

In February 2007 to help healthcare professionals understand the impact health literacy was having on patient health and safety, TJC released the white paper, *What Did My Doctor Say?: Improving Health Literacy to Protect Patient Safety*. This paper highlighted the need for healthcare organizations to establish a safe patient environment across the care continuum through effective communication (TJC, 2007). TJC requires accredited health institutions to identify and address each patient's health knowledge needs and encourages healthcare providers to partner with patients through information exchange and active patient participation in planning and executing healthcare.

In 2008, some hospitals began to voluntarily report the results of the Hospital Consumer Assessment of Healthcare Providers and Systems (HCACPS) (CMS, 2011). In June 2010, the ANA's House of Delegates passed the resolution "moving from health literacy toward patient literacy," making health literacy a major initiative for ANA (Trossman, 2010). Also in 2010, the Patient Protection and Affordability Act began using the HCACPS as a measure to calculate provider payments in the Hospital Value-Based Purchasing Program effective in 2012 (CMS, 2011). Communication with the patient is reflected in HCACPS allowing the patient's interpretation of care to determine provider reimbursement.

On January 1, 2013, under the Physician Fee Schedule (PFS), Medicare began to pay for two Current Procedural Terminology (CPT) codes (99495 and 99496) that are used to report physician or qualifying nonphysician practitioner care transition management services for a patient following a discharge from: (1) an inpatient acute-care hospital, (2) an inpatient psychiatric hospital, (3) a long-term care hospital, (4) a skilled nursing facility, (5) an inpatient rehabilitation facility, (6) a hospital outpatient observation or partial hospitalization, or (7) a partial hospitalization at a community mental health center (CMS, March 2016). The main task in care transitions is making sure the patient is knowledgeable and successful in the management of his or her health status. Patient education is the main tool used in this stage of healthcare. Successful patient education can decrease the amount of resources expended, whereas less than optimal patient education can place patients in a cycle of recidivism that becomes very dangerous to their health and finances (CMS, December 2016).

Today, even with all the technological advances that society has achieved, especially in healthcare, the common task of communicating health information to the patient still remains virtually undefined. Although patient education is the legal responsibility of every licensed healthcare provider (Kraut, 1981), it remains an unstructured and usually ill-planned exchange that occurs in most patient-provider interactions (Clark and Gong, 2000; Clark et al., 1997; Makoul, 2003). This lack of focus on patient education has perpetuated the previously discussed phenomenon of health illiteracy, which has had devastating effects on human health across the globe.

The literature reveals that patients want more information from their healthcare providers (Boberg et al., 2003; Jenkins et al., 2001). Providing patient information is a crucial part of clinical practice and directly influences a patient's satisfaction, compliance, self-management, independence, understanding, and overall health outcomes (Falvo, 2004; Redman, 2004). The goal of patient education is to increase patients' knowledge and understanding of their health. Patient teaching can only be effective if the patient learns through meaningful dialogue and understands the information provided (Sorrell, 2006). Deficits in the distribution of patient information could be related to the provider underestimating a patient's needs and misjudging the patient's level of satisfaction and comfort with the information offered (Makoul et al.,1995). Replacing provider's assumptions with good educational skills can empower patients with the knowledge and understanding needed to meet their health goals.

Ethics of Patient Education

Bioethics champions the patient's right to choice through informed consent (Knapp, 2006). Sullivan (2003) states that bioethics shifts the focus of healthcare toward patient-centeredness and challenges providers to expand their area of concern beyond patients' physical bodies to patients' lives and values (Sullivan, 2003). Patient education falls under the umbrella of bioethics, although it is addressed only peripherally through the doctrine of informed consent (Falvo, 2004). Poviders have an ethical responsibility to ensure patients are effectively educated throughout their hospitalization, so that they can be prepared to care for self and don't return to the care center again for the same issue. Spending the last 20 minutes of a hospital stay discussing the patient's illness and follow up care, is not adequate patient education. Handing the patient materials to read on his way home does not help empower the patient with information that will help them control and improve their helth status. (NurseJournal.org, 2019).

Withholding or distorting patient information can be considered unethical and dangerous as it may lead to patient harm (Fallowfield and Jenkins, 1999; Redman, 2008). Falvo (2004) identifies the ethical responsibility that healthcare providers have in delivering information to patients in a fair, honest, and unbiased manner. Breach of this duty is noted as a paternalistic approach to healthcare delivery where providers assume control in the patient-provider relationship and use "because-I-said-so" reasoning with their patients. Limiting the information a patient receives can cultivate patient dependency on healthcare providers, which can lead to personal gain for some healthcare providers (Falvo, 2004).

Changes in Healthcare Impact Patient Education

Although the clinical encounter may still be very informative for healthcare providers, as a result of 20th-century advances in biomedical technology, the main sources of patient health information are retrieved from lab tests and machines versus a verbal exchange with the patient (Roter et al., 2001). Roter et al. (2001) maintain that patient education has moved from its narrow medical illness-related approach to patient education toward a broader paradigm of personal empowerment and disease prevention. Studies focused on patient education for preventive health behaviors suggest that patient education positively contributes to disease prevention (Mullen et al., 1997). Studies have shown that patient education can increase patient knowledge (Devine, 2003; Glasson et al., 2006; Guevara et al., 2003). Patient safety (Lorenzen et al., 2008; Ratzan, 2007), and health outcomes improve with a progression in patients' health knowledge (Devine, 2003; Glasson et al., 2006; Guevara et al., 2003). Although this new paradigm is a sign that healthcare is moving in the right direction, patient education remains an ill-defined yet mandated licensed healthcare provider responsibility. To enable constructive dialogue, a platform of shared knowledge is required between provider and patient (Makoul, 2003).

The literature reveals that the health-knowledge needs of patients are not valued as much as their physical needs (Friberg et al., 2006). Most licensed healthcare providers are not specifically reimbursed for patient education (Miller et al.,1997). Lack of reimbursement affects the allocation of resources and the attention needed to make a significant impact on the successful health education of patients (Wagner et al., 2001). A lack of fiscal remuneration for patient education could be seen as an unspoken statement of the worth of patient education, implying that it is not a valuable duty in the hierarchy of healthcare.

Care Transitions

THE NEED TO ACT

People are living longer, they are living sicker, and they are living sicker longer (Cromie, 2006; DeGregori, 2003). Research shows that more than 100 million residents of the United States (30 to 40% of the population) have one or more chronic diseases, and of that group, more than half are not receiving the appropriate care (Glasgow et al., 2002). Two-thirds of the Medicare population has more than four chronic illnesses (Wagner, 2004). In 2003, more than 95% of all Medicare expenditures were spent on the treatment of chronic illnesses, such as diabetes, congestive heart failure, and chronic obstructive pulmonary disease (Wagner, 2004). Chronic illnesses caused 40 million sick days in 2004, which resulted in more than $1 billion dollars lost in productivity (Wagner, 2004). The alarming increase in the number of individuals with chronic illness, along with the increase in life expectancy, will place even more challenges on our already overtaxed healthcare system (Glasgow et al., 2002). A shift toward increasing the autonomy of healthcare consumers could provide needed relief for our overburdened healthcare system.

People may be living longer, but they do not feel any better: Patient education is something that "can make life better for people" (Tattersall, 1995, p. 375). Personal adaptation and psychological adjustment are paramount for a chronically ill patient (Cooper et al., 2001). Through knowledge, a patient can cope with poor health and altered health states, which can improve health outcomes and enhance quality of life (Cooper et al., 2001). Providers make treatment decisions with the intent of improving patients' health and lives, but quality of life should be defined individually and determined by the patient (Tattersall, 1995). Personal definitions of quality of life are seen every day in patients' actions of protest. Patients protest to assert their definition of quality of life as the basis for managing their health status. Refusing treatment or not participating in a therapeutic treatment regimen may been seen as a patient's assertion of his or her definition of quality of life.

For example, a diabetic patient detouring from the treatment course by choosing to regularly consume a piece of pie or cake may be asserting their personal definition and values about quality of life. In many instances, such individuals are fully aware of the damage that will ensue as a result of their actions.

The Cost of 102-Year-Old Nana's Care

Nana is the oldest living person in our little town. Nana is an Asian-American female who is 102 years old. She lives at the nursing home in town. Nana ambulates with a walker and is able to assist with her activities of daily living. She was diagnosed with diabetes mellitus at the age of 42. Nana has a history of hypertension, hyperlipidemia, peripheral vascular disease, and depression. At the age of 50, Nana had a total hysterectomy because she was diagnosed with and treated for cervical cancer. Nana also has osteoporosis and has developed a pronounced curvature in her spine. Nana ingests 14 different oral medications and has 2 injections administered daily. At the age of 71, Nana had a stroke that left her with residual right-sided weakness and poor vision. Since that time, Nana has required 24-hour-a-day nursing assistance (31) years and has been a resident of Willow Woods Long-Term Care Facility for 30 years. The estimated cost of caring for and maintaining Nana's health since her first diagnosed chronic illness is around $4 to 4.5 million dollars. Willow Woods is proud of their famous resident Nana, the town's only centenarian.

Health spending in the United States topped the overall national market increase by 3% per year, resulting in a growth from 13% of gross domestic product (GDP) in 2009 to 18% in 2019 (Mikulic, M. (2019). U.S. Health Expenditure as Percent of GDP 1960–2019). According to Spann, the estimated annual price tag of low health literacy is estimated to be as much as 238 billion dollars. Dollars in health literacy are spent because patients do not understand the communications and expectations of their healthcare providers (Spann, S. (2016). The incredible costs of low health literacy).

Providers Need to Know How to Teach

Parker et al. (2003) call for someone to take on the responsibility of educating the patient and for payers to reimburse patient educators for their educational services. Many Americans with the greatest healthcare needs, including the elderly, have the least capacity to understand and independently act upon the healthcare information that has been provided to them (Bayliss et al., 2007). Healthcare providers' methods of communication often do not facilitate the patient's ability to receive, process, and use health information (Miller et al., 1997; Vernon et al., 2007).

A study of 182 diabetic patients and 63 primary care physicians found that the physicians did not feel they possessed the skills needed to adequately adjust information for each patient's educational needs (Seligman et al., 2005). To help providers learn how to deliver health information, the Ad Hoc Committee on Health Literacy of the AMA proposed the inclusion of health literacy education in the training of healthcare providers (American Medical Association Ad Hoc Committee on Health Literacy for the Council on Scientific Affairs, 1999). A 2007 study published in the *American Journal of Healthy Behavior* reviewed the use of standardized patients, lay people hired to act as patients, in the training of medical residents in patient education or patient-provider communication. The study found the use of standardized patients in patient education training to be an effective teaching technique for healthcare providers (Manning and Kripalani, 2007). Harper et al. (2007) advocate for a task-oriented approach to teaching healthcare providers how to accommodate for health literacy; their approach outlines that the task be completed in a simple manner, such as, "use plain language" and "check for understanding" (Harper et al., 2007). Good patient education serves as a foundation for quality care (Tattersall, 1995). Patient education may cost more in advance, but ultimately, the cost of care will be less, and money will be saved (Tattersall, 1995). Tailored patient education can increase medical advice adherence, improve self-management of chronic disease, and increase the likelihood of better health outcomes (Billek-Sawhney and Reicherter, 2005).

Patient Education Methods

There are a myriad of methods used in patient education in clinical practice. The most common methods used for patient education are one-on-one instruction, lecture, demonstration, handouts or instructional booklets, videos, provider referenced online materials. Pictographs, pictorial symbols of a word or phrase, can be helpful to healthcare professionals in relaying information and improving the education of their patients (Greenburg, 2001). In a 1998 study and a follow-up study in 2000, researchers found that using pictographs increased subjects' recall of verbal information from 17% to 85%. (Houts et al., 1998; Houts et al., 2000).

Teaching products may assist in instructing patients, but the need for a patient educator to help the patient receive and process information is vital. Multimedia, including video education, has the potential to complement a patient educator's teaching efforts, especially for patients who are visual learners (Davis et al., 1998; Doak et al., 1995; Yancey et al., 1995). For example, a randomized heart failure study of 76 patients revealed that video education can assist in patient learning of symptom management, but concluded that video education should be used as an adjunct to in-person education (Albert et al., 2007). Hill et al. (2009), found that in the population over 60 years of age, video instruction was slightly more effective for prevention of falls than an instruction book. Although multiple patient educational tools are available to complement a patient educator's instructional efforts, one major limitation of these tools is their inability to accommodate the unique needs and informational receptivity of the person receiving the information. Patients need a healthcare provider to help them as they try to grasp new information and merge it with their personal frame of reference for real-world application (Redman, 2004).

Cultural competence in healthcare is an issue that frequents the agendas of various professional and political groups (Dogra et al., 2009) because cultural competencies address disparities in healthcare (Kleinman and Benson, 2006). The concept of cultural competence has been difficult to apply in the healthcare setting (Kleinman and Benson, 2006). Individual patient-centered education, however, moves beyond cultural influence to personal well-being.

Summary

- Health literacy needs to move from being disease oriented to being patient oriented.
- There is a need to transition patient education from the global standardized health information one-size-fits-all models to an individually focused effort tailored specifically for the specific patient.
- Although healthcare providers may be a valuable source of information, more training may be needed to be effective in patient education.
- Today, even with all the technological advances that society has achieved, especially in healthcare, the common task of communicating health information to patients remains virtually undefined.
- Patient teaching can only be effective if the patient learns through meaningful dialogue and understands the information provided.
- People are living longer, they are living sicker, and they are living sicker longer. A shift toward increasing the autonomy of healthcare consumers could provide needed relief for our loaded healthcare system.
- Teaching products may assist in instructing patients, but the need for a patient educator to help the patient receive and process information is vital.
- Patients need a healthcare provider to help them as they try to mentally grasp and then merge the new information into their personal frame of reference for real-world application.

CHAPTER 3

Education Theory

In healthcare, patient education can save quality of life, empower patients with choices, and decrease the cost of care. Patients educated about their health are better able to understand and manage their own health and medical care throughout their lives (Marcus, 2014). To truly meet patient needs, providers should understand how to communicate with patients using educational principles and theory. This chapter will review the educational principles and theory that can help healthcare providers empower their patient with knowledge.

Two overarching theoretical educational frameworks serve to support the strategies used in the art and science of human learning: pedagogy and andragogy. These theoretical structures are thought to cover the process of educating humans across their lifespan. Francis Bacon believed in two types of learning: learning in children and learning in adults. Bacon spoke of pedagogy as the framing of morality. Adult learning, in Bacon's writings, is closely associated with religious beliefs and challenging mental faculties. Regarding adult learning, Bacon maintained that we cannot teach people, we can only help them in their learning (Bacon, 1893). A review of the theories of pedagogy and andragogy can help a patient educator in approaching the initial stages of cultivating health knowledge in a patient.

Pedagogy

Pedagogy is derived from the Greek words *paidi* (meaning child) and *agogus* (meaning leader of). In Latin, the term *pedagogue* means *teacher*. Hence, *pedagogy* means the art and science of teaching children (Knowles et al., 2005). The pedagogic model of education is a set of principles that are based on assumptions of teaching and learning that evolved between the 7th and 12th centuries in the monastic and cathedral schools of Europe through their experiences teaching young boys (Knowles et al., 2005). These traditional pedagogic curricula were grounded in social and political values, free of student ideology and discernment (Alexander, 2004). Didactic information, deemed socially relevant, was instilled into students through subject-oriented content. Pragmatism and conformity were cornerstones of the traditional curricula (Alexander, 2004).

In a pedagogic model, the learners' "need to know" is predetermined for them by the teacher (Knowles, 1984). The teacher is the axis of control for what students will be taught, how it will be taught, and what will constitute successful educational achievement (Hiemstra and Sisco, 1990). Learning is teacher planned, delivered, and directed in pedagogy. The student role is one of submissiveness and dependence on the teacher in the learning quest (Hiemstra and Sisco, 1990). External motivators such as grades, teacher approval, and parental pressure are familiar tools used in pedagogic learning.

Why Is Taylor's Mom Delivering His Newspapers?

Taylor, the local paperboy, is in the ninth grade at St. Joseph's Middle School. Recently, several town locals have spotted Taylor's mother, Joanie, delivering more papers on Taylor's paper route than Taylor. According to Ms. Haddie, Taylor and Joanie's next-door neighbor, Joanie is having Taylor spend more time on his algebra homework. Apparently, Taylor is having great difficulty grasping the basics of algebra. St. Joesph's Middle School is a feeder school to St. Patrick's High School, which is a college preparatory school; Taylor has to make a "C" or better in ninth-grade grade algebra to qualify for admission into St. Patrick's. Taylor would prefer to take geometry because he did so well in it in the eighth grade, but to meet St. Patrick's admission prerequisites, he must successfully complete ninth-grade algebra.

EXPERT SUPPORT FOR ACTION

Traditional pedagogic curricula are grounded in social and political values, free of student ideology and discernment (Alexander, 2004). Didactic information deemed relevant is instilled into students through subject-oriented content (Alexander, 2004). In a pedagogic model, the learners' "need to know" is predetermined for them by the teacher (Knowles, 1984). The teacher controls what will be taught, how it will be taught, and what will constitute successful educational achievement (Hiemstra and Sisco, 1990).

In the 19th century, when secular schools were established in the United States, the pedagogic model was used because it was the only known model of education (Knowles et al., 2005). Pedagogical assumptions served as the theoretical framework for all educational efforts, including for higher education that involved adults. For multiple generations, adults were taught using the same methodology as children. After World War I, assumptions about adult learning started to emerge (Knowles et al., 2005). These assumptions began to establish a foundation that would progress into an educational philosophy and would ultimately form the theoretical framework of andragogy.

Andragogy

The term *andragogy* comes from the Latin word *andr*, which means man. Andragogy is the art and science of helping adults learn (Knowles et al., 2005). American adult educator Malcolm Knowles may be known as the father of andragogy, but he was not the first to coin the phrase. In 1833, the term *andragogy* was first introduced by a German schoolteacher, Alexander Kapp, who used the word to describe the educational theory of the Greek philosopher Plato (Knowles et al., 2005). A few years later, German philosopher Johan Friedrich Herbart expressed his opposition to the use of the term *andragogy* in the description of the great Plato, which caused the term to fall out of favor and to disappear for nearly 100 years. In 1921, the term resurfaced when it was used by Eugen Rosenstock-Huessy, a German social scientist who expressed the opinion that adult learners require a special teaching approach based on the unique methodology and philosophy of andragogy (Knowles et al., 2005). In 1951, Heinrich Hanselmann, a Swiss psychiatrist, published the book *Andragogy: Nature, Possibilities, and Boundaries of Adult Education*, which focused on the re-education of adults. In 1956, 1957, and 1959, publications in academic and secular literary works thrust the term *andragogy* into mainstream usage (Knowles et al. 2005).

In 1950, Malcolm Knowles published his first book, *Informal Adult Education*, which explicated the concept that adults learn best in informal, comfortable, flexible, nonthreatening settings. The groundbreaking work of Malcolm Knowles' theory of andragogy has helped add definition and focus to the art and science of adult learning. However, his work also sparked controversy in the world of academia.

Malcolm Knowles' assumptions were derived from studies done on the adult learner, primarily by psychologists Piaget and Erikson (Knowles, 1973, 1980). He proposed that as individuals mature into adults, their concept of self changes the manner in which they approach learning. Knowles' theory has six assumptions about the adult learner. Each of these assumptions easily translates into patient education in the healthcare setting.

According to Knowles (1975), adult learners:

1. Need to know why they need to learn something
2. Are self-directed and maintain responsibility for decisions and life events

3. Bring a growing reservoir of experience that serves as a resource for learning in the educational activity

4. Have a readiness to learn things they need to know to manage their life and real situations in their various social roles

5. Are life-centered in their orientation to learning

6. Are more responsive to internal motivators than external motivators

In response to these assumptions, Knowles calls for educators to:

1. Set a cooperative learning climate

2. Create mechanisms for mutual planning

3. Arrange for an analysis of learner needs and interests

4. Establish learning objectives based on the identified learners' needs and interests

5. Design sequential activities to achieve the objectives

6. Execute the design by selecting varied methods, materials, and resources

7. Evaluate the quality of the learning experience while diagnosing additional learning needs

In andragogic methodology, the instructor shifts from the pedagogic role of the source of information to that of a facilitator, an expert resource who helps guide the learner toward knowledge (Knowles et al., 2005). Educator and learner work together to meet mutually identified learning objectives. The learner helps establish the direction of instruction by communicating personally perceived knowledge needs. Knowles used a five-point scale from low to high for learner self-evaluations (Knowles, 1975). In andragogy, the learner is self-directed, actively seeking and moving toward knowledge. The employment of various resources and methodologies assists the instructor in guiding the learner toward desired information (Knowles, 1950, 1975). Andragogy theory advocates for the educator-learner activity to be inclusive of learner values, life experience, and learner-identified needs in establishing the foundational structure for adult education.

How 48-Year-Old Jim Educates Himself About Diabetes

Jim, a local plumber, is a 48-year-old Caucasian male who has been diagnosed with diabetes mellitus. Jim has been attending local diabetes education classes and reading information published by the American Diabetes Association. Jim has progressed through grieving for the loss of his health and has accepted his diagnosis. Jim feels he needs to take control of his disease and is ready to resume power over his life. He has sought out information online and is actively participating in his diabetes class. Jim states that he is feeling stronger because he now understands how to carry out his daily care and the reason these actions are needed. Because Jim has assumed responsibility over his care, his blood glucose levels have remained stable within the targeted range established by his primary-care physician.

Understanding pedagogical and andragogical methodology can help establish capacity and context in education activities. Both philosophies bring forth various responses of teacher and learner, while offering external and internal influences affecting knowledge-gain in conventional education. Although both pedagogical and andragogical principles can be applied to any learning scenario, the unique influences encountered in the healthcare setting present a need to specifically focus on health education.

Medagogy

Patients who misunderstand what their healthcare providers are trying to communicate to them can suffer devastating, and potentially fatal, consequences (Osborne, 2005). The treasure chest of assumptions from pedagogy and andragogy offers a good footing on the path to teaching patients and accommodating their learning needs. Challenges encountered by patient education activities cannot be met solely through customary academic approaches. It is necessary for patient educators to understand that each patient is a unique learner. The challenge is determining how healthcare providers can best structure information so each patient can receive it, understand it, remember it, and apply it.

Medagogy offers a theoretical foundation that healthcare providers can use to construct a defined, methodical approach to patient education. Medagogy examines the process of patients' knowledge construction, acquisition, and proliferation as they move through the healthcare system (Stewart, 2009). Each healthcare provider serves as a source of health knowledge, while each patient serves as a source of self-knowledge. Both provider and patient have an active role in contributing to the progression of each other's knowledge. Together provider and patient can forger a health plan that is reflective of patient values and health care goals.

It is a daily challenge for healthcare providers to educate people whose health statuses are virtually consuming their every thought. The charge of helping someone make a mental connection with critical information in a time of crisis is rare in traditional education but a normal occurrence in healthcare (Friberg et al., 2007; McCabe, 2004). Information from the healthcare provider has bearing on the health, life, and welfare of the consumer of healthcare services: the patient. Information from the patient influences cost of care, inclusion of personal values, self-perceived ability, and health outcomes (Friberg et al., 2007). Whether it is for preventive intercession or a reaction to insult or lifestyle, teaching a patient involves circumstances that are not regularly encountered in traditional education (Falvo, 2004; Friberg et al., 2007; Redman, 2004).

When laypersons (patients) access the healthcare system, they are entitled to receive information regarding their health status and options for healthcare. Patients may present with health ranging from excellent to critical. To maximize resources and assist patients in attaining their health goals, providers must communicate via information exchange with patients; this is patient education. Medagogy focuses on the art and science of patient education by providing a conceptual framework for understanding the patient in the learning process (Stewart, 2009). The conceptual framework for medagogy is discussed in detail in Section 4.

Significance to Healthcare

Patient teaching is a core component of professional practice for healthcare providers (Boyd et al., 1998). Patient education has been referred to as the "essence of nursing" (London, 1999, p. 7). Healthcare providers serve as the perfect medium to help patients gain health independence, provide appropriate self-management, enhance treatment adherence, and improve overall health status (Friberg et al., 2007; Henderson, 2002). Although healthcare providers are strategically positioned to assume the role of patient educator, not all providers have been adequately taught how to educate patients and their families. Luker and Caress (1988) targeted a large population of healthcare providers when they boldly asserted, "nurses are not good teachers" (p. 714). The inadequate performance of any healthcare professional as an educator may result from a lack of training in the skills of teaching or educating (Chang and Kelly, 2007; Luker and Caress, 1988; Marcus, 2014). The lack of provider training in the art of teaching only amplifies the problem of addressing patient knowledge because the student in the healthcare setting is a patient.

The healthcare student (i.e., the patient) deals with multiple barriers to learning. Examples of possible barriers to patient learning include pain, fear of the unknown, separation from support systems such as family and friends, unfamiliar surroundings, and problems at home (e.g., childcare concerns and fiscal impact of health insult). The illness of the patient-student, not to mention the potentially fatal errors in self-care that can occur if patient learning is not achieved, makes patient education a challenge (Gabbay et al., 2000).

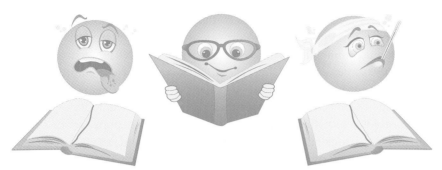

Fig. 3.1   Three patient-students are reading. Two of the students are ill and distracted, whereas the healthy student is involved in reading the book he is holding. The figure serves to display the learning barrier that physical illness can present.

Healthcare environments establish a teaching climate that does not parallel traditional academic settings. Figure 3.1 is a visual representation of two ill students and one healthy student. Many time patient don't even know when the provider is delivering important health information.

In healthcare, the patient educator has to make sure the patient can receive the information delivered. The patient's health status can interfere with reception of information, potentially acting as a barrier to learning and ultimately forestalling health-promotion (Gabbay et al., 2000).

World leaders who define quality in medical practice understand the need for patients to be knowledgeable about their health status and whether healthcare services are needed. The World Health Organization and the European Commission reports highlight that effective communication is critical to understanding health information (Stableford and Mettger, 2007). The Institute of Medicine (IOM), the Agency for Healthcare Research and Quality, and the Health Association Libraries Section, a component of the Medical Library Association, have all produced reports that stress the need for clear, congruent, legitimate information for patients (Stableford and Mettger, 2007).

The practice of teaching healthcare providers to communicate information and evaluate patient understanding has not been a research priority for all healthcare professionals, but it is needed to address the major concern of the lack of health literacy (Major and Homes, 2007). Health literacy expert Greenburg (2001) notes that patients need to get their health information delivered according to learning principles and educational theories. Greenburg (2001) also calls for the availability of health educators to whom healthcare providers can refer patients for education. The patient educator would help the patient understand their health status and treatment. Greenburg (2001) suggests that patient educators be used to teach healthcare information based on the individual patient's needs. According to Erlen (2004), healthcare providers are in a unique position to provide the needed interpretation and information accommodations for patients. Greenburg (2001) refers to patient education as a new and evolving specialty that could become embedded into holistic patient care. Through good patient education, patients acquire the knowledge they need to cope with their disease, which can reduce mortality and morbidity and enhance a patient's quality of life (Cooper et al., 2001). A patient's personal adaptation or psychological adjustment and acceptance should be of paramount concern to healthcare providers (Cooper et al., 2001).

The teaching styles of some healthcare providers create learning barriers (Tattersall, 1995), whereas other barriers such as fear and pain are common in healthcare (Smith, 2011; Bastable, 2006). Patient-provider communication can improve through evaluating patient comprehension and instructing providers on how to teach patients (Paasche-Orlow et al., 2006). People have varying learning styles and different literacy levels. Patient education must be designed to accommodate each individual's educational and cultural diversities and abilities (Curry et al., 2005; Kurashige, 2008). According to Bastable et al. (2006) and Parikh et al. (1996), learning is an intricate, difficult, and demanding skill that needs to occur in a conducive environment. In 1999, five categories for influencing the development and improvement of patient education were identified (Deccache and Aujoulat, 2001).

1. Healthcare organization
2. Professional value
3. Healthcare policy
4. Evidence-based practice
5. Training and methodologic support

Training and methodologic support refers to the education of healthcare providers in the multidimensional process of human learning (i.e., training providers to be educators). In an attempt to address the health-knowledge needs of healthcare consumers, the Organization of Patient Educators (OPE) released a course that trains healthcare providers in andragogy and pedagogy, laws of learning, behavioral theories, and the theory of medagogy. The OPE certifies healthcare providers who complete the patient educator course, implement a patient teaching plan, and pass an intensive examination as Certified Patient Educators (CPEs). The information taught in the course is used every day in the practices of CPEs.

In the Centers for Medicare and Medicaid 9th scope of work's pilot-care transitions, the Louisiana Quality Initiative Organization (QIO) used the medagogy framework. After pilot employees of the CMS were trained and credentialed by OPE, the medagogy model was used for all patient education. The unique patient-oriented approach of medagogy was successfully used to meet the care-transitions benchmarks of CMS. In 2011, the QIO, which used medagogy, was acknowledged by CMS as the nation's most innovative healthcare pilot program for their successful work in care transitions. (Griggs, 2011; Johannessen, 2010).

Summary

- There are two overarching theoretical educational frameworks that serve to support the strategies used in the art and science of human learning: pedagogy and andragogy.
- *Pedagogy* means the art and science of teaching children.
- In pedagogy, learning is teacher planned, delivered, and directed. The student role is one of submissiveness and dependence on the teacher in the learning quest.
- *Andragogy* is the art and science of helping adults learn.
- In 1950, Malcolm Knowles published his first book, *Informal Adult Education*, which explicated the concept that adults learn best in informal, comfortable, flexible, and nonthreatening settings.
- The treasure chest of assumptions from pedagogy and andragogy offer a good footing on the path to teaching patients and accommodating their learning needs.
- It is necessary for patient educators to understand each patient is a unique learner.
- Medagogy offers a theoretical foundation that healthcare providers can use to construct a defined, methodical approach to patient education.
- Medagogy examines the process of patients' knowledge construction, acquisition, and proliferation as they move through the healthcare system. Both provider and learner have an active role in contributing to the progression of each other's knowledge.
- The charge of helping someone make a mental connection with critical information in a time of crisis is rare in education but is a normal occurrence in healthcare.

- The healthcare student (i.e., the patient) deals with multiple barriers to learning. Examples of possible barriers to patient learning include pain, fear of the unknown, separation from support systems such as family and friends, unfamiliar surroundings, and problems at home with childcare.

- In healthcare, the patient educator has to ensure the patient can receive the information delivered.

- The practice of teaching healthcare providers to communicate information and evaluate patient understanding has not been a research priority for all healthcare professionals, but it is needed to address the major concern of the lack of health literacy.

- The teaching styles of some healthcare providers create learning barriers, whereas other barriers like fear and pain are common.

- In an attempt to address the health knowledge needs of healthcare consumers, the OPE released a course that trains healthcare providers in andragogy and pedagogy, laws of learning, behavioral theories, and the theory of medagogy. The OPE certifies healthcare providers who complete the patient educator course, implement a patient teaching plan, and pass an intensive examination to become a CPE.

- Medagogy offers the prospect of bringing the skill of patient education into an organized, interdisciplinary healthcare model used to educate each patient so his or her health-literacy needs and healthcare goals can be adequately addressed.

Section I Summary

In healthcare, the patient-provider relationship offers unique educational opportunities that are unlike the conditions that exist in any other institution. Each patient is a unique student with one-of-a-kind qualities and needs. Often, patients do not receive the information they need from healthcare providers. An accurate understanding of health-related information is needed for patients to partner with providers and for providers to partner with patients to achieve optimal healthcare goals and favorable outcomes. Healthcare providers need to diligently plan and carefully articulate the information patients need to be involved and active in their healthcare (Redman, 2003). Patients need to assert their healthcare goals and knowledge, which will help them assume their rightful position in the planning and management of their treatment. Good patient education serves as a foundation for quality care (Tattersall, 1995). Patient education may cost more in advance, but ultimately the cost of care will be less, and money will be saved (Tattersall, 1995). Patient education is a basic duty of healthcare providers. Successful patient education is a gift of knowledge that empowers individuals and families. Patients have the right to understand their health conditions so that they can make informed decisions and be in control of their healthcare (US Department of Health and Human Services, 1999). Medagogy offers the prospect of bringing the skill of patient education into an organized, interdisciplinary healthcare model to be used to educate each patient so his or her health-literacy needs and healthcare goals can be adequately addressed.

Effective Teaching and Learning

CHAPTER 4

Information Exchange

Information, although an essential element in the healthcare provider-patient relationship, can also be an empowering tool. This section will focus on definitions for teaching and learning as they relate to patient education and knowledge attainment. Teaching methodologies and theories both assert beliefs regarding what happens in the teaching and learning process, although these methodologies and theories are usually associated with traditional educational settings (i.e., schools and colleges). This section is intended to expose the reader to information that can aid the healthcare provider and patient educator in mastering the teaching and learning process in the healthcare setting.

Patient-Provider Exchange of Information

Possessing information can be a personal source of enlightenment regarding choices and potential opportunities, whereas a lack of knowledge can cloud the decision-making process. People function within the limits of their knowledge. A lack of information can be detrimental to the quality of choices that are made (Hirsch, 1988). To completely capture the process of information delivery between healthcare provider and patient, the information exchange must be explored from provider to patient and patient to provider. A narrow focus has long governed patient education and the patient's assumed gain of understanding from provider-delivered information (Mordiffi et al., 2003). Patient education has focused on the provider's role in sharing their knowledge with the goal of moving the patient forward in their healthcare (Boyde et al., 2009). Although providers educating patients may intend to increase patient understanding, simultaneously they need to recognize their position as pupils of their patients in the provider-patient information exchange process (Safran et al., 1998; Weiner et al., 2005). Providers need to gain an understanding from the information they receive from the their patients (Hahn, 2009; Weiner et al., 2005). This includes learning about the intricacies of the patients' personal lives.

Educator and learner roles constantly reverse throughout provider-patient communication interactions. Just as healthcare decisions are made from the information the patient receives from the provider, the provider also learns valuable information from the patient (Hahn, 2009). Providers use the details of the information the patient shares to assist in the construction and formulation of a treatment plan. The more insight the provider has, the more patient-specific the provider can be when rendering treatment options and participating in treatment planning (Boyde et al., 2009; Wakefield and Jorm, 2009; Weiner et al., 2005). The flow of information between the patient and healthcare provider is a fluid dynamic that perpetually stimulates change and action through choice for both receivers (Hahn, 2009).

In healthcare, there is a need for the patient-learner to receive instruction as well as to educate the provider to their personal experiences, values, and goals (Epstein et al., 2005; Hahn, 2009; Leonard and Wilijer, 2007). Likewise, the need exists for the healthcare provider to instruct the patient regarding knowledge of human health, healthy behaviors, and health options, as they simultaneously receive instruction from the patient. The more personal knowledge the provider gains about a patient, the better the communication between the provider and the patient will be (Mordiffi et al., 2003). Shared information between provider and patient will result in a progressive experience that will allow each to directly exert influence in treatment planning (Epstein et al., 2005; Leonard and Wilijer, 2007; Tang and Lansky, 2005). Allowing personal influence increases the likelihood of including individual preferences and values while moving toward optimal health (Kaufman 2008; Shaw et al., 2009).

Knowledge is a source of power. Traditionally, the provider has assumed power in the patient-provider relationship (Epstein et al., 2005; Leonard and Wilijer, 2007; Walford and Alberti, 1985). Influence in treatment has been limited to the healthcare provider's assertions and assumptions (Leonard and Wilijer, 2007; Mordiffi et al., 2003). Although the healthcare provider brings expert health knowledge to the provider-patient relationship, too often what the patient brings to this relationship is overlooked, ignored, or assumed (Boyde et al., 2009; Mordiffi et al., 2003). To ensure all facts and influencers in care are addressed, patient and provider should both be seen as an expert. The patient is the expert of self, whereas the provider is the expert of healthcare. Both the patient and the provider hold vital information, knowledge, and skill needed to obtain and maintain health. Lack of acknowledgment of personal knowledge brought to the relationship can delay and or impair health progress in the patient. Therefore, it is reasonable to acknowledge that the teacher and learner roles constantly shift between the patient and the provider. For example, when learning about the patient's history, health goals, and personal resources, the patient would assume the teacher/expert role and the provider would be the learner/novice. Conversely, when describing assessment findings and the possible diagnosis, the provider would assume the role of teacher/expert and the patient would be the learner/ novice. Constant role exchange as learner/novice and educator/expert occurs throughout the healthcare relationship between provider and patient.

Every learner is unique, and so is every patient. Each patient presents with his or her own definition of health as it relates to self. Each patient is presenting in a healthcare setting or participating in a healthcare information exchange because of their desire for a goal related to their health. As a healthcare provider, it is imperative that the patient's reason for health-education access, whether face to face or digital, is determined. The patient's impetus for access is the driver for the patient to seek help. If the patient is respectfully included in treatment planning, both patient and provider can learn a great deal from each other while executing an effective, individualized treatment plan that could achieve optimal health outcomes.

Span of Influence

The literature supports the relationship between knowledge and power (Bishop, 2009; Hutchinson et al., 2009; Rumsey et al., 2003; Simonton, 1985). This means that patients with more information have a greater ability to influence their healthcare. The span of influence is directly and indirectly related to the understanding of information associated with a given situation. Figures 4.1 and 4.2 visually display the relationship between knowledge gain and span of influence.

As the span of influence increases, the amount of direct effect a person can have over a situation enlarges. The wider the span of influence is, the greater the personal influence a person can exert in the planning and delivery of their healthcare treatment. A large span of influence may be present but not used if a patient does not claim and exercise the power associated with their span of influence (Bishop, 2009; Longtin et al., 2010; Rumsey et al., 2003). The personal power connected with the span of influence must be asserted to influence the patient's treatment plan.

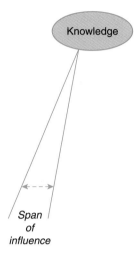

Fig. 4.1   Span of influence. Span of influence is the area between the angled lines. The degree of area represented in the span of influence is related to corresponding knowledge. © Melissa N. Stewart.

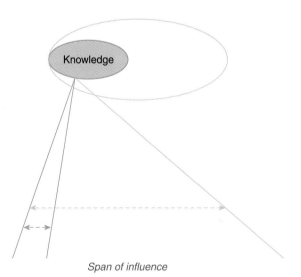

Fig. 4.2   Expanded span of influence. Increased knowledge increases the span of influence. The figure depicts a positive relationship between expansion of knowledge and increased span of influence. © Melissa N. Stewart.

Lack of Communication With Provider Resulted in Patient Ignoring Physician Advice

Roger is a 52-year-old Asian male who entertains the community at public events as a musician. Roger admittedly tries to avoid healthcare providers as much as possible. As a child, Roger had to visit his pediatrician and therapist often because of leg braces he had to wear to correct genu varum, bow legs. He recalls his obstinacy to the leg-brace therapy and the lack of control he had in whether or not to use the prescribed treatment. This early interaction with the healthcare field left Roger with an overwhelming feeling of powerlessness as a patient. His impression of healthcare providers in early childhood has influenced his interaction with healthcare providers throughout his life. As an adult, Roger avoids engaging in the healthcare system. However, when he is forced to access healthcare, Roger answers questions quickly and concisely. Roger tries to get a solution to what he perceives as a health issue in the quickest, least personal way. The healthcare provider offers a solution, and Roger decides after the visit if he will or will not adhere to the provider's suggestion. Because Roger grew up feeling his opinion was not valued by the provider, he has made healthcare an impersonal business transaction. Laughingly, Roger stated that he has a better relationship with the self-serve gas station he uses than he does with his primary care provider. Roger firmly believes that his primary care provider does not even know he is a person, let alone his patient. The lack of relationship and effective communication between healthcare provider and patient prompted Roger to miss his follow-up visits after his last hospital stay for pneumonia. This interruption in the treatment course caused Roger's condition to exacerbate and resulted in re-admission to the hospital only 20 days after his discharge. Roger lost time at work, and his insurance had to pay for an avoidable hospital readmission.

EXPERT SUPPORT FOR ACTION

Fear and pain are common in healthcare (Perry 2006). Add to the learning environment the factors that patients may experience like illness, emotions (i.e., fear, anger, insecurity, and sorrow), financial insult, pain, chaos, urgency, and more, it is easy to see how learning can become even more challenging (Levinson et al., 2000; Rolls et al., 1994). Fear, lack of control, and grieving for loss of health are all emotions that patients are likely to experience in healthcare (Jervey 2001; Mitchell et al., 2008).

Teaching

The teaching-learning process is a dynamic and complex activity that continues to impress and puzzle expert educators. From the science of behavior to the evolving field of neurocognitive science, the teaching and learning process has yet to be completely understood (Wlodkowski, 2008). Although science may not ever completely grasp all that occurs in the teaching and learning process, there are many elements that are generally accepted as integral to the process. Teaching, one of the oldest professions in the world, focuses on knowledge exchange. Plato's scholarly interactions with his students helped to establish teaching methodology that framed knowledge for generations beyond the protégés at his feet. Religious orders, such as monastics, committed their lives to improving society through education (Feldman and McPhee, 2008). Political equality movements used education to limit social distortion and remove barriers (Mondale and Patton, 2001; Nasaw, 1997). Through all the changes that have occurred in education, one constant has remained: knowledge is power. Knowledge offers control and enlightenment to the beholder. As Francis Bacon affirmed, knowledge serves as an intellectual map that helps as one chooses the right path (Price, 1893). The art and science of teaching focuses on the act of delivering information designed to enlighten the receiver through knowledge acquisition and increased personal wisdom (Alexander, 2004; Knowles et al., 2005). Pring (2004) asserts that to teach is to engage intentionally in those activities that bring about learning.

Academia has evolved into the presently accepted setting for teaching and learning. Although teaching takes place in various settings, school in today's society is the traditional setting where teaching, instruction, and training are routinely performed. Public schools with mandated attendance have helped to condition members of society to automatically assume the role of student upon entry into an academic setting (Mondale and Patton, 2001; Nasaw, 1979). School settings are universally accepted as a resource for information and a destination for improved knowledge.

Internet

Today education is limitless, as it has progressed from the brick-and-mortar schoolhouse to the unlimited access available with internet connectivity. According to a 2001 Pew internet and American Life Project, students are no longer poring over pages for information after hours of searching a library; the convenience of the internet has placed information just a click away. The internet provides a venue to conveniently access research for papers or schoolwork (Lenhart et al., 2001). Instant messaging and e-mail communication with peers and instructors can provide students with homework assistance in minutes (Lenhart et al., 2001). Websites can serve as sources of information for students or projects for learning through website construction (Lenhart et al., 2001). Computer technology with internet access removes many traditional limitations and boundaries in education, offering powerful educational resources for the learners who are proficient in their utilization (Chang et al., 2004). Unfortunately, the population most affected by health decline and chronic illness, those who are 65 years of age and older, are caught in the "digital divide," either because of limited access or lack of internet and computer knowledge (Campbell 2008; Chang et al., 2004; Kaye, 2009). The commonly experienced effects of aging, such as decline in vision, hearing, and dexterity, only add to the geriatric population's challenge in accessing advanced technology (Czaja and Lee, 2007). A 2009 report revealed that the geratric population is beginning to access the internet more than they have in the past (Jones and Fox, 2009). Although this news is promising, there is still much work that needs to be done in providing the geriatric population with internet health resources (Jones and Fox, 2009).

Centeredness of Information and Instruction

In healthcare, the patient is the heart and soul of any and every task and obligation. The same centeredness should carry over into patient education. One major duty of an educator is the identification of information that is prudent and beneficial for the learner to know. In the classroom, the teacher serves as the courier of information that faculty, administration, and academic standards have deemed prudent and beneficial for the learner to know. However, in healthcare, the task of identifying prudent and beneficial information for the learner is not as planned and constructed. Healthcare has traditionally focused on the physical ailments and disorders of the body. However, to meet the patient's health needs, healthcare providers must concentrate on addressing the patient's knowledge and learning needs along with physical issues, health-promotion, and prevention (Myers and Pelino, 2009).

Traditionally, the patient-education encounter is educator centered. The information that is to be taught is prioritized through the provider's knowledge of the patient's health status and a myriad of assumptions regarding the patient's life and values (Boyde et al., 2009). These assumptions could be clarified and validated with the patient, but usually are not. This type of educator-centered instruction occurs when educators deliver information that they think the learner needs (Mordiffi et al., 2003). Educator-centered instruction constructs information according to provider-oriented needs rather than patient-oriented needs and reinforces the traditional segmenting of patients into disease or health states; information delivery should instead be formatted totally for the patient. Patients should be taught holistically with information that reflects who they are and where they are in their personal health (Boyde et al., 2009). Information should be tailored toward that individual's "thumbprint" or one-of-a-kind knowledge needs (Boyde et al., 2009; Oliver et al., 2001).

Prefabricated patient-education products and third-party manufactured presentations contain disease-oriented information and serve as examples of educator-centered instruction because the individual patient is not included in the formation of these products. Producers of these products work from assumptions about the potential receiver's learning needs, priorities, and values and their foundational level of understanding new information. Individuality and personalization are removed from most conventional disease-oriented patient education materials. This is not to say that these products should not be used in healthcare; they can be used in a learner-centered teaching plan if they are complemented with a patient educator who frames the information to match the patient's life (Boyde et al., 2009; Mordiffi et al., 2003). To be truly learner centered, all instruction and teaching materials should be personalized to meet each individual patient's learning and knowledge needs (Bull et al.,1999; Falvo, 2004; Kyngas, 2003).

To address a patient's knowledge and learning needs in healthcare, an educator should construct a learner-centered plan for teaching. Learner-centered instruction focuses on issues and matters that are important to the learner. Ideally, the learner would help establish the prioritization of material to be taught by communicating his or her desired knowledge. Values, health goals, finances, and many more factors help influence the manner in which the patient receives, understands, and prioritizes information. Understanding the multitude of socioeconomic influences that patients experience can help a provider respect the choices patients ultimately make from the information the provider offers (Hahn, 2009).

Healthcare offers a unique situation in that the knowledge needed may not be apparent to the learner. This lack of knowing is related to the healthcare provider's knowledge of health and treatment, that is, the provider's healthcare expertise. The provider's expert knowledge is imperative in planning and prioritizing patient education. Learner-centered teaching in healthcare focuses all plans for education on the learner's needs, resources, individual knowledge, and health status (Hahn, 2009; Redman, 2006). If the learner does not recognize his learning deficits because of his lack of healthcare expertise, then the expert with that knowledge, the provider, must expose the learner to the information he lacks. The expert should be sensitive to the knowledge deficits that the patient might be experiencing. Learner-centered teaching is planned through the partnering of provider and patient (Bensing, 2000; Boyde et al., 2009). This partnership offers an opportunity to construct a personalized teaching plan that is unique to each and every patient.

Situational Centeredness

As previously noted, healthcare is not a traditional learning setting. Healthcare by its very nature creates this singular educational environment. Although learner-centered instruction is desirable, it is important to acknowledge that it is not always appropriate in the healthcare setting. The unique milieu of healthcare frequently requires situational-centered instruction because the challenges of illness, injury, and emergencies often leave the learner's situation in a volatile flux (Epstein et al., 2005). There are instances where healthcare decisions must be made within moments; in these instances, information has to be relayed as quickly as possible (Bensing, 2000). As a patient's health status stabilizes, information can then shift into a learner-centered focus (Bensing, 2000). Healthcare environments require perpetual assessment on the part of the healthcare educator to know when the patient needs situation-centered information or learner-centered information. Centeredness of the information must be appropriate for the presenting health state (Bensing, 2000).

This present change in situation demands a strong commitment on the part of the provider to ensure that the patient's rights are always maintained as the priority (Falvo, 2004; Rankin and Stallings, 2001; Redman, 2007). As discussed previously, patients have the right to make healthcare decisions. The patient's right to information allows the patient to exert control over healthcare decisions, while still honoring the patient's right to receive what he or she wants from the healthcare provided (Rankin et al., 2005).

How the Provider Transitioned Patient Education to Focus on Emergency Need

An example of transitioning the centeredness of patient education can be seen in the example of Steve, a 33-year-old Caucasian who is a chef at the fancy restaurant in town. Steve had a recent stay in the local acute hospital when he became an injury victim from a rock that was thrown by a neighbor's lawn mower. The rock hit and lodged in Steve's left eye, and he was rushed to the local emergency room. Steve and his family were immediately offered information regarding Steve's status and his need for surgery. Because of the sensitivity of the situation and the need to act swiftly, information was clear, concise, and direct. The information was centered according to the situation, which required immediate attention, the insult state. Steve went through his surgery and remained an inpatient for 2 days.

Continued on following page

While Steve was an inpatient, his patient education from the unit staff focused on things he needed to know as he transitioned to home, such as:

- Medications
- Follow-up appointments
- Infection control methods
- Dressing change procedure
- Signs and symptoms of infection

Information was also inclusive of Steve's voiced concerns, issues he felt were important:

- Who to call if he has a health-related issue
- What to do if he forgets to take his medication
- When can he go back to his normal routine
- And most of all, when can he return to work

Every member of the staff added some piece of knowledge to Steve's health understanding, but before assuming Steve felt ready to do for himself, the hospitalist, Dr. Badu, asked Steve how he felt about his ability to carry out his care independently. Dr Badu's focus on Steve's comfort with assuming his self care duties, also the staff's dedication to making sure Steve received the information he needed and wanted, motivated Dr. Badu to offer Steve patient education in a more patient-centered approach than the patient education he had received pre-surgery in the emergency room.

EXPERT SUPPORT FOR ACTION

The patient provides his or her expert knowledge of self, including, but not limited to, personal values, an experiential base related to disease expression, personal needs, cultural beliefs related to health and illnesses, and desired outcomes (Leonard and Wilijer, 2007; Mordiffi et al., 2003; Shaw et al., 2009). Without the information of self that the patient brings to the relationship, the treatment is at risk for misdiagnosis, misappropriation of resources, and mismanagement of health (Collins et al., 2004; Swanson, 2007). The skills and knowledge from both the self and the health expert are necessary for the formation of an effective treatment plan that will achieve optimal health outcomes (Epstein et al., 2005).

Transmitting and Recieving Information

Although educators can deliver information, they do not possess power over knowledge acquisition; they cannot make someone learn (Ormrod, 2008). Likewise, the receiver or student does not completely control the reception and retention of information (Jensen, 2000) because the entire learning process is dependent on many variables. For the teaching effort to be effective, the information or content has to make a connection with the receiver. Educators attempt to match the delivery method so the receiver's reception is improved, and long-term storage of information is probable (Jensen, 2000; Ormrod, 2008).

Summary

Information is a powerful tool used in the healthcare provider-patient relationship. This section focused on teaching and learning definitions in patient knowledge attainment. Although an increase in patient understanding may be the intention of patient education, the provider needs to recognize his or her position as a pupil of the patient and his or her personal life intricacies in the provider-patient information exchange process.

Educator and learner roles constantly reverse throughout provider-patient communication interactions.

The more personal knowledge of the patient that is gained by the provider, the better the communication between the provider and the patient.

Knowledge is a source of power. In the provider-patient relationship, power has traditionally been assumed by the provider too often, and what the patient brings to this relationship is overlooked, ignored, or assumed.

In healthcare, the heart and soul of any and every task and obligation is to the patient. The same centeredness should carry over into patient education.

Provider-centered instruction constructs information according to provider-oriented needs versus patient-oriented needs.

Prefabricated patient-education products and third-party manufactured presentations contain disease-oriented information and serve as examples of educator-centered instruction because the individual patient is not included in the formation of these products.

To be truly learner centered, all instruction and teaching materials should be personalized to meet each independent patient's learning and knowledge needs.

If the learner does not recognize his or her learning deficits because of a lack of healthcare expertise, then the expert with that knowledge, the provider, must expose the learner to the information needed.

Often in emergency situations instruction is limited to what needs to be shared initiate emergency treatment.

CHAPTER 5

The Science and Theories of Learning

Learning involves the act of receiving and storing information delivered for future access. Hirsch (1988) identifies knowledge as a network of information possessed by the learner that empowers the learner to obtain, process, and store new information. A logical intellectual connection must occur with the information that the educator is offering for learning to transpire (Hess and Tate, 1991; Rice and Okun, 1994). For example, a student who does not know numbers cannot learn geometry. A baseline knowledge of numbers must be present for the student to grasp basic concepts of geometry. For students to learn geometry, they must know numbers and the order in which they fall so they can appreciate the value of each number. The lack of the foundational knowledge in this example removes the opportunity for the intended connection of known information to newly acquired information (Santrock, 2008: Zull, 2006). Without the foundational information, the new information may be remembered, but there is no depth and fluidity with foundational basics, meaning there is no solid understanding (Ormrod, 2008; Zull, 2006). The student is missing the reasoning or the "why" of the new information.

A foundation of knowledge provides a site for additional information on which to build. For learning to occur, information must have a logical order to enable the brain to receive, process, and store the information (Noddings, 2006). Much like a building structure, the more solid the foundation, the more weight or knowledge can be added. Without a foundation, the information will have nothing solid to stand on; therefore it will not procure a permanent place in the brain. The logical order of information helps the learner sort, label, and catalog information for future retrieval (Pring, 2004; Rice and Okun, 1994). A healthy foundation allows previous knowledge to be accessible when information is acquire into proper placement and sequence in the brain. Logical order helps to simplify assimilation and the mental storage of new information for the receiver (Kessels, 2003). An example of logical order is 1, 2, 3, 4, 5 or A, B, C; whereas, 4, 1, 3, 5, 2 or C, A, B would represent an illogical order or no order.

Instructional Methodology for Optimal Learning

The magnitude of influence that information bears in the provider-patient relationship makes delivery of information a task that should be seen as a high priority. To prepare patient information so it can be well received could help to ensure that patients have a solid foundation of information. This in turn can allow a patient to make an informed decision, which ultimately affords the patient a better opportunity to control the path of his or her healthcare. Planning and preparing patient information, just as a teacher plans and prepares student information, offers an opportunity for healthcare providers to capitalize on proven academic techniques that can improve the possibility that the receiver—the patient—is successful in understanding the information delivered (Atherton, 2009; Ormrod, 2008; Sousa, 2006). Off-the-cuff delivery and/or information dispersed in the process of an assessment and/or treatment provides an unstable situation for learning to be successful.

In academia, educators choose content that students need to know along with the method of delivery for the information. The educator's goal in choosing the method of delivery should be to use methods that promote learning, best engage the learner, and facilitate the learner's mental connections that promote understanding (Sousa, 2006). Selecting a method of delivery in healthcare could, for example, be choosing between a lecture and a demonstration. It would benefit the provider to know that a lecture on how to do a fingerstick for glucose monitoring would not be as effective as watching a demonstration of someone performing the task (Sousa, 2006). According to Atherton (2009), a lecture results in 5% mental retention after 24 hours versus a demonstration, which has a 30% retention rate. Immediate use of learned information can also boost one's retention rate up to 90% (Ormrod, 2008; Sousa, 2006).

Packaging information for delivery can present a challenge for educators, especially in healthcare. Information should be delivered in a way that allows learners to best receive, process, and store the information (Ormrod, 2008). According to Pring (2004), regardless of the method of delivery chosen to communicate the information to the learner, all teaching activities should have the following in common:

- Intention to influence knowledge through learning
- Connection between what is presented and what is to be learned
- Connection between what is taught and the learner's presenting knowledge

The best method of delivery of information is dependent on what is best for the patient. The educator must also choose methods that correlate with the educator's personal skills and proficiencies. Lack of educator competency in a teaching skill may serve as interference in the patient's assimilation and storage of information (Feldman and McPhee, 2008; Ormrod, 2008). Therefore, the selection of methodology for information delivery should be learner centered while being educator mastered.

Currently in patient education, most instruction is done one-to-one at bedside or chair side with the patient, and occasionally in classes with other patients. If a patient needs assistance with care or needs support, then family or significant others may also be included in patient-learning sessions. One-on-one instruction offers the opportunity for the educator to construct and deliver the information for individual patients and meet their personal needs. Too often in healthcare, the education patients receive ends up being either a presentation that is repetitively done for every patient with a certain disease condition, or an off-the-cuff "oh, and you need to know" delivery.

Many times, the one-on-one teaching sessions are at the convenience of the educator and do not coincide with optimal timing nor a learning environment for the patient. An example of educator versus patient timing is diabetic nutritional teaching after a tired patient finishes a 2-hour physical therapy session late in the afternoon in a rehabilitation hospital. The timing is perfect for the dietitian's schedule as she closes out her workday. However, it is less than optimal for the patient who is physically and mentally tired. However, preplanning and asking the patient what time works best for his/her learning could help both the provider and patient get the education sessions in sync (Redman, 2006).

Sometimes learning opportunities present themselves, and, if ignored, the teachable moment has passed. These teachable moments are excellent at revealing where the patient is in their desire for knowledge (Falvo, 2004). These moments can initiate a fruitful learning experience as they offer the educator insight into the patient's knowledge priorities, allowing the educator to answer and address extraneous information that may have been overlooked because of its relevance only to that particular patient. These serendipitous teaching moments also allow the educator to display a commitment to meeting the patient's personal knowledge needs by immediately providing attention to the patient's informational request (Redman, 2006). The information that is exchanged in these sessions should be included in the patient's teaching plan and become part of the patient's learning history (Falvo, 2004; Rankin et al., 2005).

Scheduled one-on-one teaching sessions can allow for the patient to add input to the direction of the teaching interaction. Educators must be open and encourage each patient to identify and share his or her self-diagnosed knowledge needs (Hahn, 2009; Tang and Lansky, 2005). Offering choices allows patients control in their education and the opportunity to insert their lifestyle, daily needs, and value system into their wellness program (Coates, 2007). Allowing personal injection of preference and interest provides an opportunity in the construction of thorough patient understanding in the pursuit of health through patient empowerment (Stone et al., 2005; Tang and Lansky, 2005).

Conscious and Unconscious Learning

Jensen (2000) noted that only 10% of learning is conscious (explicit), whereas the remaining 90% is unconscious (implicit) (Shanks, 2010). The brain is such an amazing organ that it initiates learning before conscious learning is initiated (Jensen, 2000). Unconscious or implicit learning absorbs information from the whole picture through the use of sights, smells, and sounds, (Jensen, 2000; Shanks, 2010). Jensen (2000) refers to implicit learning as learning through the body. Data begins to be internalized on an unconscious level even before the first piece of planned information is formally

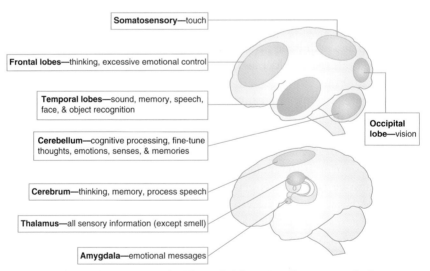

Fig. 5.1 **Areas of the brain used with implicit learning (Sousa, 2006).** The various areas of the brain that are involved in information processing and storage with implicit learning are shown.

delivered (Jensen, 2000). Figure 5.1 displays the areas of the brain that are used with implicit learning (Sousa, 2006). Knowing the amazing abilities of the brain in learning can help educators as they plan educational sessions. Knowing that the learning environment, from sounds to tactile sensations, will have a part in the memory of the learner acknowledging and planning his or her healthcare education can help the educator better prepare so that the intended message is received and reinforced. Educators should strive to establish an optimal learning situation, so they can maximize what is captured in the conscious (explicit) 10% of learning. A screaming, crying patient in the hall can negatively impact a message focused on teaching a preoperative patient effective pain control. The visual (seeing a person crying) and auditory (the sounds of screaming and crying) senses are stimulated in this example. The emotions are also triggered as the patient is concerned with approaching surgery and most likely fearful of imminent postoperative pain. Unless a written form accompanies the verbal information delivered, retention might not occur because of hyperstimulation of senses triggering conscious attention on the sensory information being received.

To ensure that the patient will learn the information intended to be communicated in a planned learning moment, the educator needs to capture the student's attention (Feldman and McPhee, 2008). Experience has taught the author that the patient educator needs to persuade or move the intended learner, the patient, into a state that is receptive to learning. Consciousness of learning, according to the author, is a voluntary state of attention, focusing on certain prescribed information. Information may be new, old, associated with, or similar to information previously learned, or refreshing already-stored information. To motivate the learner to move into a consciousness for learning, the teacher or educator must gain the learner's interest by leading the learner to an awareness, which can occur in several different ways (Feldman and McPhee, 2008). Movement into a learning consciousness happens after engagement occurs. Engagement includes mental and physical awareness and appeal. The attraction mentally and physically enables concentration on the information being delivered. Engagement prioritizes information so that it mentally and physically limits personal attention toward other environmental options, while centering attention on the information being conveyed. Once the receiver is engaged with the deliverer, then a concentrated effort on learning can occur.

To help engage a person, one might try a provocative question—stimulating interest in what is being said, while at the same time stimulating thinking—as the learner mentally positions his or her stance while pulling forward known history related to the question (Feldman and McPhee, 2008).

Staggering statements like "40% to 80% of what a healthcare professional says is forgotten almost immediately" (Kessels, 2003) and profound or famous quotes, such as "we will either find a way or make one," likewise offer the opportunity to capture the learner's attention (The Motivating Tape Company, 2000). A story of a problem, empirical data that support possible outcomes, or conveying personal experience can serve as an attention getter for learners (Feldman and McPhee, 2008).

Engaging a learner also involves a physical concerted effort to show the learner that he or she is your present focus. Physically, the educator needs to get on the same physical level, facing the learner eye-to-eye and heart-to-heart (Boothman, 2002). A person who is in front of you and talking directly to you while looking you in the eye can grab your attention. Educators need to talk with compassion, concern, and confidence as they teach. The patient educator needs to humanize the information, personalizing it for patients so they can easily fit it into their individual worlds. Casual conversation and active listening on the part of the educator can help in the extraction of information from the patient that can be used in the personalization of information that is presented. The more that is known about the person, the more the information can be personalized (Boothman, 2002).

In constructing and planning what information needs to be delivered, knowing the patient's level of knowledge on a topic is beneficial. Simple discussion with probing questions can help an educator to gain insight into a patient's knowledge of a condition. For example, the healthcare provider might ask, "Tell me about congestive heart failure. What is it?" Another method that might be used is "test by discussion," which offers social interaction while providing relevant personal information. Each individual will be different in how receptive they are to the time it takes them to understand, or to discern if they understand. The celebration of human learning is the uniqueness of each individual in the learning process. Patience and skillful reframing of information for patient clarity can be very beneficial attributes in a patient educator. Once a patient's understanding of information is gained, then the caregiver can determine how to communicate more information to him or her.

Learning Domains

In the 1950s, American educational psychologist Benjamin Bloom identified learning domains, which include six levels of human thought that differ in complexity (Bloom, 1956). Each level of thought is dependent on the preceding level for successful accomplishment (Ormrod, 2008). Bloom's work illustrates the mental construction that human thought must complete to reach higher levels of understanding (Krathwohl et al., 1964). Autonomy and personal definition are achievable with stair-step maneuvering of knowledge up through the learning domains.

Bloom organized his cognitive levels into a taxonomy that many educators use in the construction of educational learning goals and objectives. Bloom's taxonomy assists educators in identifying where students need to be in their cognitive mastery of the information, while providing direction in increasing the complexity of knowledge. In 2001, Anderson and colleagues revised Bloom's taxonomy to incorporate theoretical advances that have been made in education. The revision transitioned the taxonomy into a two-dimensional model, including six cognitive levels and four types of knowledge. Anderson et al. (2001) identified types of knowledge as factual, conceptual, procedural, and metacognitive. Bloom's taxonomy can help educators better plan and strategically target their teaching efforts to assist students in their mastery of knowledge. Table 5.1 offers a comparison of Bloom's work to the 2001 revision.

The table parallels the original cognitive levels identified by Bloom to the revised cognitive levels of Anderson and colleagues. The third column lists the four types of knowledge identified by Anderson and colleagues.

In the teaching of patients, understanding the levels of knowledge can help the patient educator in moving the patient from a level of remember to a level of apply.

TABLE 5.1 ▨ **Comparison of Bloom's Original Work to Revised Works**

Bloom	*Anderson and Colleagues*	
Cognitive Levels	**Revised Cognitive Levels**	**Types of Knowledge**
Knowledge	Remember	Factual
Comprehension	Understand	Conceptual
Application	Apply	Procedural
Analysis	Analyze	Metacognitive
Synthesis	Evaluate	
Evaluation	Create	

Data from: Anderson, L.W., Krathwohl, D.R., Airsian, P.W., Cruikshank, K.A., Mayer, R.E., Pintrich, P.R., ... Wittrock, M.C. (Eds.). (2001). *A taxonomy for learning, teaching, and assessment: A revision of Bloom's taxonomy of educational objectives.* New York: Longman.
Bloom, B. (1956). *Taxonomy of educational objectives: The classification of educational goals.* New York, NY: Longman Publishing Group.

A Simple Demonstration Showed How to Avoid Aggravating Peripheral Vascular Disease on the Job

Mr. Boudreaux is a 67-year-old Cajun fisherman who has peripheral vascular disease (PVD). Mr. Boudreaux has been told for years that he needs to elevate his feet. Mr. Boudreaux can repeat past instruction without error. He fully complies with the limitations of no crossing legs and no elastic binding socks or tight underwear or pants. Mr. Boudreaux demonstrates that he remembers and understands the information. Recently, Mr. Boudreaux was assigned to a new post at his job. The new position requires Mr. Boudreaux to be in a harness that wraps around his waist and inner thighs and lifts him in the air. After two days in the new position Mr. Boudreaux was experiencing such leg pain and swelling that he had to see the company nurse, Donna. Even though Mr. Boudreaux has been a model patient in hearing and following his providers' advice, he did not grasp the reason for the treatment recommendations he was given. Mr. Boudreaux could not apply the treatment rule of "avoid any constriction of circulation in your legs" to the new harness he was wearing for his new position. Mr. Boudreaux was not able to see the harness as a means of constricting circulation in his legs. Helping Mr. Boudreaux master the ability to apply this rule independently should be the provider's focus for his education. Recognizing Mr. Boudreaux's inability to apply the treatment instruction, avoid circulatory constriction, impelled Donna to explain to Mr. Boudreaux the PVD disease process. Donna then reviewed the symptoms that can occur, such as leg pain and swelling, while correlating the symptoms back to Mr. Boudreaux's presenting complaints. Mr. Boudreaux explained that he understood what happened. Frustrated he went on to explain that he did not know how he would be able to always recognize things that could cause this event to happen again. Donna took an oblong balloon and blew it up half way, then she pushed on one end forcing the air to move toward the other end. She then pushed on the opposite end forcing air to the other side. She asked Mr. Boudreaux, "do you see how easily the air moves in the direction I want it to?" Mr. Boudreaux confirmed that he did. She handed the balloon to Mr. Boudreaux and had him manipulate the balloon, forcing air to shift side-to-side like she had done. Then Donna applied pressure to the center of the balloon and asked Mr. Boudreaux to shift the air to the other side. Mr. Boudreaux applied pressure and stated "I don't want to pop it though" as he made the air shift to the other side as Donna directed. Donna then stated, "it wasn't as easy to make the air move, was it"? "No," stated Mr. Boudreaux, "not while you are pinching it." Donna then compared the balloon with Mr. Boudreaux's leg. She went on to state that the pinching is a form of constriction. Just as the air shifted to one side and stayed on that side while she was pinching the balloon, the same thing happens when blood flow in the legs has something pinching or constricting the flow; the blood will stay on one side and swell because it is too difficult for the body to push the blood through the pinched area. Mr. Boudreaux said, "Oh, so I need to think of my legs like a balloon." "Absolutely, you are correct," answered nurse Donna. "Now you will always remember that anything that tightly grabs an area of your leg can cause the blood flow to be restricted, and that will cause swelling. So yes, Mr. Boudreaux, think of your legs as balloons and avoid anything that causes 'pinching.'"

EXPERT SUPPORT FOR ACTION

Without foundational information, the new information may be remembered, but there is no depth and fluidity with foundational basics, meaning there is no solid understanding only a basic familiarity (Ormrod, 2008; Zull, 2006). Aristotle (2009) asserts that within the understanding of "why" lies reason, which provides an insight or wisdom that can be used beyond the immediate intended utility. Understanding "why" helps establish a foundational rationale, which can be an asset in treatment decisions for the provider and the patient (Tokarz, 2009). When behavior modification is hoped for, then providing a "why" upfront for the desired behavior change can ease the discomfort of confusion associated with lack of access to, and therefore, lack of understanding of the full picture (Jensen, 2000; Redman, 2007).

Teaching and learning are intensely personal activities; not all teachers are the same, and more importantly, not all learners are the same. For teachers to be able to convey the desired information to the pupil, they must be able to meet each learner's distinct needs (Brookfield, 2006). Educators should attempt to personalize the design and delivery of information to accomplish this objective (Avillion, 2009).

Learning Styles

Knowing a person's learning style can help the educator tailor the delivery of information to the learner's preferred (and most effective) learning style. There are three types of perceptual processing learning styles: visual, tactile, and auditory (Avillion, 2009). According to Minninger (1997), approximately 55% of the general population are visual learners. Visual learners use the sense of sight to facilitate their mental ingestion of information. Seeing information helps to aid visual learners in processing and retaining it. Visual learners prefer to see illustrations, graphics, color, and even the instructor (Avillion, 2009).

The second most common learning style is tactile, which is also referred to as kinesthetic (Minninger, 1997). An estimated 30% of the population favors the kinesthetic learning style (Minninger, 1997). This type of learner is commonly referred to as a "doer." Learners that are doers are "hands on" learners who are best able to process information through experiencing the information via action or feeling. Physical movement, as well as handling and manipulating items can assist the tactile learner in knowledge absorption (Avillion, 2009).

Verbal and auditory learning is the third learning style. It is favored by 15% of the population (Minninger, 1997). Verbal learners need to speak or read aloud and to discuss or explain information in an effort to process the knowledge through auditory stimuli (Avillion, 2009). Auditory learners best receive and remember information that is heard. These learners may appear as if they are not interested in what is being communicated, when in fact they are actively listening (Avillion, 2009).

Material delivered according to a personal learning style can help the learner receive and process the information with ease, while increasing the likelihood for overall success in the learner's educational experience (Anonymous, 2009; Feldman and McPhee, 2008; Costa et al., 2007). Unfortunately, knowledge of a person's learning style is not always available. Many healthcare admission forms ask patients their preference for receiving information, but people do not always know what learning style they favor or what learning styles could yield their best personal results. An answer to the question does not necessarily mean the delivery mode chosen by the patient has accurately identified their learning style.

A mixed approach of teaching can help an educator tap into all learning preferences in information delivery (Jensen, 2000). This approach incorporates all teaching/learning styles and can aid in delivery through exposing the student to information via each learning sense. Using teaching methods that accommodate multiple learning styles ensure that the learner's personal learning preference is included in delivery (Avillion, 2009). If, indeed, not all learning styles can be used because of the nature of the material to be taught, the teaching setting, or the teaching method, then when planning information delivery, targeting the most common learning styles can offer a greater chance of success.

Teach About High Cholestrol Using Props and Mixed Teaching Methods

Physician assistant (PA) Jan, plans to teach patient Mike about his cholesterol. On hospital admittance, Mike, a 32-year-old welder identified reading as his favorite way to receive information. Jan noticed that Mike had a crossword puzzle book in his hand. Because Mike listed "building projects" as a hobby and appeared very inquisitive about his treatment, Jan had a printout of material she planned to review, one for her and one for Mike, as well as props, including a piece of water hose, blue cotton balls, red cotton balls, and a crossword puzzle to use in their scheduled training session. Jan verbally reviewed with Mike the information they would cover in their session that day. Jan then began to read from the handout sheet while Mike followed along on his sheet. After reading the handout, Jan then began to use her props, the hose and colored cotton balls, to visually show Mike the impact of plaque (red cotton balls) buildup in the arteries (hose). Jan even had Mike put the red cotton balls in the hose. Jan used the blue and red cotton balls to show the desired relationship of good and bad cholesterol. After many laughs and questions, Mike laughed as he stated that he never knew his garden hose could help save his life and that now he really understood how important his cholesterol is to his health. Jan then gave Mike a crossword puzzle that used all the information they had reviewed that day and told Mike he had homework. Mike briefly glanced at the puzzle and said he would have it done before she came back to see him again. Jan gathered her props and told Mike that she would return in a couple of hours to check on him and retrieve his homework. Mike appeared to have enjoyed the instruction, while Jan was able to communicate very important information. Jan's ability to use mixed teaching methods, tapping into all learning styles, was evident by the following:

- Auditory: discussion, verbal exchange
- Kinesthetic: patient physically putting cotton ball in hose, laughing, and completing a crossword puzzle
- Visual: use of props, including colored cotton balls, hose, and a crossword puzzle

EXPERT SUPPORT FOR ACTION

Studies show that individualized instructions increase comprehension and memory more effectively than standardized instructions (Morrow et al., 2005; Robinson et al., 2008).There are three types of perceptual processing learning styles: visual, tactile, and auditory (Avillion, 2009). Healthcare providers need to present information in a manner that each patient can understand, recall, and use in their lives and healthcare choices (Stableford and Mettger, 2007). A mixed approach of teaching can help an educator tap into all learning preferences in information delivery (Jensen, 2000). Using teaching methods that accommodate multiple learning styles ensures that the learner's personal learning preference is included in delivery (Avillion, 2009).

Overlap Between Teaching and Learning

Once information is received, the work of knowing/learning begins (Brookfield, 2006; Jones, 2000). Teachers can present information, but the assimilation of the material offered is the work of the student or receiver. Just as the teacher has been charged with the task of teaching, the receiver or student, bears the responsibility of accepting and internalizing that information, ultimately resulting in learning the information (Demetriou and Raftopoulos, 2005). Recognizing the inherent interdependent relationship of the concepts, teach and learn, along with the fact that both teacher and learner have to work to make knowledge delivery and assimilation occur, it is easy to conclude that the process of knowledge gained through instruction is a shared function between the teacher and the learner.

Learning Theories

In learning, knowledge or an understanding is gained by study, instruction, or experience. Learning is a science. From neuron firing to schemata filing, many theories have tried to explain the process of learning, but just as no two fingerprints are the same, such is each individual experience in learning. At best, words can only serve to point out commonalities of beliefs associated with the process of learning. In an attempt to provide a conceptual framework to the process of traditional education, multiple theories have evolved. Theories of learning attempt to explain how learning occurs (Knowles et al., 2005).

Three prominent theoretical views hold sway in education regarding how learning occurs and the factors that influence learning: behaviorism, cognitivism, and constructionism. Although some educators are committed to one primary philosophy and choose to label themselves as a member and a practicing party of a particular theoretical belief, the process of learning is so uniquely personal that a broad knowledge of theoretical perspectives and their complements to the field of education can better serve an educator (Feldman and McPhee, 2008). It is never clear, when humans are involved, whether one recipe can suit all (Falvo, 2004; Redman, 2006). Therefore, it is the author's belief that patient educators should not conform to a single educational theory but should instead understand the underlying dogma and amalgamate parts of theories, which can complement the personal practice of the patient educator. The following theories are considered influences of medagogy.

Behaviorism

Behaviorists define learning as a change in behavior as a result of experience and the creation of habits and see the mind metaphorically as an empty container (Feldman and McPhee, 2008). Behaviorists believe that human learning can only be explained through observable behaviors (Skinner, 1974; Thorndike, 1911). According to behaviorists, people act only as they are conditioned; behaviorists believe that learning is only induced through external forces via conditioning (Baum, 2005; Skinner, 1991).

This theory asserts that all human behavior, from emotions to reasoning, can be explained and predicted through associations between external stimulations and the response to these stimuli (Feldman and McPhee, 2008; Hilgard, 1988; Pavlov, 1927; Skinner, 1974, 1991; Thorndike, 1911). Reflexive and automatic associations are known as classical conditioning

(Pavlov, 1927; Watson, 1930). In the healthcare setting, it is normal for patients to become anxious when they see a provider, a phenomenon commonly referred to as the "white coat syndrome" (Engler, 2005; Harlan, 2007; Kerr, 2008). The white coat syndrome is the result of negative stimulation or experiences recurring in a healthcare setting. For example, a child receiving a shot every time they visit a physician will eventually associate the physician with shots. In time, the mere mention of the physician may stimulate a sense of fear as seen in Figure 5.2.

Edward Thorndike authored three behaviorism laws, which fall under the umbrella of his connectionism theory. According to connectionism, learning is the result of associations formed between stimuli and responses (S-R) (Ormrod, 2008; Thorndike, 1911, 1932; Thorndike et al., 1928). Strong associations or "habits" can be strengthened or weakened depending on character, positive or negative, and the regularity of exposure associated with S-R pairings

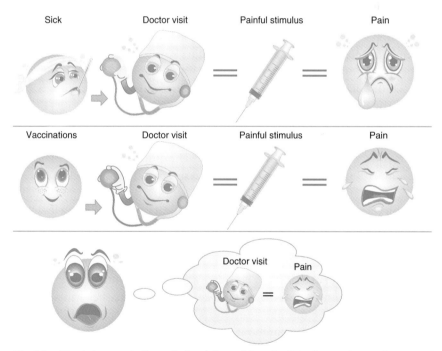

Fig. 5.2 Mental association of physician with pain. The figure shows the mental associations that can be formed from a consistent introduction of a painful stimulus, an injection, during a doctor's office visit. In health or illness, if a painful stimulus is consistently introduced, then a mental association between a doctor's visit and pain can occur. Once the association is established, just the thought of a doctor visit can trigger thoughts of pain.

(Lefrancois, 1995; Kearsley, 2009; Ormrod, 2008). As Figure 5.2 shows, the regular stimulus of a shot during physician visits yields a negative response of pain, that eventually creates a mental association of visit equates to pain. Thorndike found that certain responses dominated others (Lefrancois, 1995; Kearsley, 2009; Thorndike, 1911, 1932; Thorndike et al., 1928). He noted that positive reinforcers directly increased the frequency of desired behavior, and discomforting or punishing responses decreased the frequency of undesired behavior (Kearsley, 2009; Ormrod, 2008). Figure 5.2 shows that fear is associated with a physician's visit because of the mental pain association. The S-R theory evolved out of trial-and-error learning, which Thorndike identified as the most basic form of learning (Thorndike, 1911, 1932; Thorndike et al., 1928).

Thorndike asserted that neural connections were formed in response to perceived stimulus and resulting response (Thorndike, 1911, 1932). He referred to the neural connections in the brain associated with the S-R pairing as "stamping in" (learning) and "stamping out" (forgetting) (Knowles et al., 2005; Ormrod, 2008; Thorndike, 1911; Thorndike et al., 1928). Thorndike recognized that humans and animals learn in like fashion, that learning is incremental, and that a person's readiness to learn is directly proportionate to the success of the learning experience (Bash, 2005; Hoare, 2006; Knowles et al., 2005). Three primary laws born from Thorndike's connectionism theory are the law of effect, the law of readiness, and the law of exercise (Bower and Hilgard, 1981; Kearsley, 1996; Merriam and Caffarella, 1991). The law of effect states that recurrence of responses is strengthened or weakened by its consequence or reward (Ormrod, 2008; Thorndike et al. 1928). The law of readiness maintains that if a sequence of responses known to yield a certain desired outcome is blocked, it will result in annoyance, which may diminish the level of desire to learn in the student (Kearsley, 1996; Knowles et al. 2005; Thorndike et al., 1928). The law of exercise asserts that S-R connections that are repeated are strengthened, while S-R connections that are not used are weakened (Bower and Hilgard, 1981; Merriam and Caffarella, 1991; Thorndike et al., 1928). Thorndike's three laws continue to exert major influence in human learning and the application of new behaviors.

Modified behavior through learning is known as operant conditioning. Operant or instrumental conditioning was coined by American psychologist B.F. Skinner (Ormrod, 2008; Skinner, 1966, 1984). He asserted that conditioning in behavior occurs because of rewards or punishments that happen in response to behavior (Ormrod, 2008; Watson, 1930). Behaviorists maintain the validity of three principles (Baum, 2005), each of which complements each other. The first principle states that predictable links exist between a stimulus and the response it yields (Pavlov, 1927; Skinner, 1974,

1991; Thorndike, 1911; Watson, 1930). The second principle contends that through study and manipulation of conditions that influence behavior, behavior can be shaped and predicted with a high degree of certainty in a specific situation (Skinner, 1974, 1991). The third principle states that varied reinforcement can strengthen or weaken learned behavior (Feldman and McPhee, 2008; Pavlov, 1927; Thorndike, 1911; Watson and Rayner, 1920). Many weight-loss programs use behaviorism to modify member behavior. In support meetings, members weigh in, and weight loss is celebrated with rewards, whereas weight gain may involve negative consequence, such as increased cost or possibly even dismissal from the program. The use of rewards and punishments helps condition or train the behavior of members to meet desired goals (Pavlov, 1927; Skinner, 1974, 1991; Thorndike, 1911; Watson, 1930).

Implications for the practice of patient education derived from the behaviorism theory center around the behaviorists' belief that knowledge is not something that exists in the mind, but instead works as a form of guidance formed from actions (Baum, 2005; Feldman and McPhee, 2008; Watson, 1930). A patient educator's awareness of conditioning through external influence and the role that reinforcement plays in learning and behavioral change can be valuable in patient teaching for lifestyle improvement. Behaviorism supports the position that positive or negative reinforcement can affect patient (pupil) motivation, which can have direct consequences in the provision of healthcare and the establishment and implementation of a treatment plan. As with the previous example in Figure 5.2, negative mental associations will need to be addressed. The patient may not want to follow up with the physician because of negative mental associations with the physician visit. An explanation of the purpose of future visits by the physician in regard to the treatment plan may help alleviate the patient's fear.

Skinner tried to explain human language using behaviorism underpinnings (Overskeid, 1995). Chomsky challenged Skinner's behavioral position with the notion that individuals choose syntax in verbal communication (Chomsky, 1959; Green, 1994). Although the cognitive processes of attention, consciousness, memory, and perception referenced here are mentioned in behaviorist theory, behaviorism does not focus on the brain's inner functions (Cognitivism, 2009; Overskeid, 1995).

Cognitivism

Cognitivism is sometimes referred to as classical theory. In the 1950s and 1960s, researchers began to investigate learning from inside the human brain, focusing on human thought. This new approach to thinking was called cognitivism, the science of the mind (Feldman and McPhee, 2008; Roland, 2008). The cognitivism paradigm distinguished a higher level of ability in the human brain versus the animal brain, claiming that the human brain is capable of a higher order processing of information (Roland, 2008). The capacity to apply logic and be rational in the processing of information exposes more of the higher level function of the human brain (Ramey, 2005; Roland, 2008). The cognitivist view of the human brain is similar to that of the central processing unit in a computer. Cognitivists believe that information enters the brain, and then human thought processes the information (Feldman and McPhee, 2008).

Swiss psychologist Jean Piaget's work in cognitive development and educational psychology made significant contributions to the theory of cognitivism. Piaget postulated that a person's interaction with the world assisted in the formation of mental concepts and the mental representation of reality (Piaget, 1954, 1967; Piotrowski, 2005). Piaget identified cognitive development in four stages: sensorimotor, preoperative, concrete operational, and formal operational (Piaget, 1954, 1967; Piotrowski, 2005; Santrock, 2007, 2008). Piaget deemed language a tool that contributes to cognitive development through exercises of personal interaction with the world (Piaget, 1954, 1967; Piotrowski, 2005; Santrock, 2008). He believed that language was directly reflective of cognitive maturity (Mayer, 1987; Piotrowski, 2005). Young children, because of immature and egocentric thought, are not concerned with external opinion. According to Piaget, with age and the mastery of logical thinking and perception, productive social interaction is achievable (Piaget, 1954, 1967; Piotrowski, 2005; Santrock, 2007, 2008). As people age, they are able to focus beyond self and become more conscious of others (Piaget, 1954, 1967).

Cognitivists believe that learning involves mental associations (Ramey, 2005). Humans possess systematic internal capabilities that are used to elucidate their surroundings (Ramey, 2005). Information received is managed according to how it meaningfully corresponds with stored data, called schema (Shuell, 1990). Schema theory, a cognitivism subtheory developed by American educational psychologist Richard R.C. Anderson, postulates that schemata are mental representations that serve to network knowledge so it can be used by the mind (Anderson and Montauge, 1984; Davis, 1991). Schemata are used by the mind to govern behavior, organize memories, interpret information or experiences, and focus attention (Armbruster, 1996; Shuell, 1990). According to this theory, recall and understanding are contingent on how new information merges with existing established schema (Anderson and Montauge, 1984; Davis, 1991).

An explanation of the variance in understanding, learning, and problem-solving capabilities among people, according to schema theory, is related to the variance in mental schemata (Shuell, 1990). Each individual's schema is individually unique because of varying personal experiences. Attachment of new information to present schema is meaning-driven per personal interpretation (Armbruster, 1996). The schema theory can clarify the cognitive differences between a novice and an expert with regard to a skill (Shuell, 1990). A novice schema does not contain the wealth of specific topic information from which an expert who has expertise on that specific topic can draw. Expert schemata contain a large well-organized body of skill, knowledge, and experience that can be quickly accessed for use. This allows the expert to intervene and maneuver more quickly and with greater precision (Durso et al., 2007). With time and practice, a novice may progress to an expert level (Durso et al., 2007).

It is imperative that educators help learners build schema and make mental connections by exposing the learner to how the new information fits with previous connections (Balota, 2004). In healthcare, patients sometimes have difficulty understanding the rationale for self-care recommendations that they are advised to carry out. Helping the patient understand what is happening within his or her body provides rationale for action that can bridge the connection to treatment options and ultimately help the patient with his or her healthcare choices. Using an analogy, such as comparing the heart function to an engine or water pump, can help the learner bridge the new information with known information (Balota, 2004).

Stage theory, another subtheory of cognitivism, focuses on the human processing of information in three stages: the input stage, the short-term memory stage, and the final stage of information consolidation in long-term memory (Balota, 2004; Durso et al., 2007; Feldman and McPhee, 2008; Stuart-Hamilton, 2006). The input stage is where information is received and becomes internalized through encoding (Balota, 2004; Stuart-Hamilton, 2006). The dual encoding effect contends that memory contains two separate interrelated systems, verbal and visual, for information processing (Feldman and McPhee, 2008).

In the second stage, information moves into the short-term memory, where it is retained for approximately 20 seconds unless it is rehearsed or grouped with meaningful information (Ross, 2006). The third and final stage includes the transition of information into long-term memory via rehearsal and/or strong emotional context (Demetriou and Raftopoulos, 2005; Feldman and McPhee, 2008; Ross, 2006; Stuart-Hamilton, 2006). Short-term memory can only hold approximately seven units or pieces of information. After that, volume capacity is reached, and the information is not retained because of short-term memory storage limitations and information overload (Feldman and McPhee, 2008; Miller, 1956; Ross, 2006; Stuart-Hamilton, 2006). To compensate for the memory's limitations, Miller (1956) developed a method called chunking. In the chunking method, bits of information are loaded into cognitive chunks that are constructed for easier transfer from short-term to long-term memory (Anderson and Montauge, 1984; Davis, 1991; Miller, 1956; Ross, 2006). This process of organizing information into chunks is known as the cognitive load theory, which is a subtheory of cognitivism.

Cognitivism is comprised of individual discoveries identified as principles that add significance to the teaching-learning process. One cognitivism principle is that meaningful information is easier to learn and remember (Demetriou and Raftopoulos, 2005; Feldman and McPhee, 2008). People learn what is of interest to them (Knowles, 1972; Knowles et al., 2005). Placement of information in presentation is relevant for memorization. The serial position effect notes that items at the beginning or end of a list are easier to learn (Feldman and McPhee, 2008; Ross, 2006; Sousa, 2006). The distributed practice effect states that practice at intervals rather than all at one time is more effective (Demetriou and Raftopoulos, 2005; Feldman and McPhee, 2008; Shuell, 1990). The principle of the distributed practice effect is used often in sports. A child learns how to play a sport. The child may show a natural aptitude for this sport. To ensure the child is successful in the development and maintenance of this sport talent, he or she has to practice. Practice does not just happen once. Instead, practice will become a routine activity for the child. Rehearsal of a sport is a strategic exercise that gradually improves performance. The principle of the distributed practice effect can be shown in medicine. For example, a patient has to begin a regimen of daily self-injections. At first, the patient may need step-by-step written instructions that can be followed while performing the injection. After multiple times of self-injecting, the instructions will no longer be needed because the information/skill will have become ingrained in the memory. The practice of the skill will improve the knowledge and performance of the procedure.

The interference effect claims that prior learning can interfere with new learning if it is not filed correctly, or is erroneous information (Anderson and Speiro, 1977; Roediger and Karpicke, 2006). The interference effect often occurs when a person is given too much listed information to remember (Roediger and Karpicke, 2006). An example of the interference effect is when a healthcare provider tells a patient four things that he or she needs to do, such as take medication for infection twice a day with meals until the bottle is empty, lose weight, return to the clinic in 3 or 4 weeks, and take the chart to the window and pay. The likelihood of the patient forgetting one of the healthcare provider's recommendations is high. The information can become confused in encoding. Unfortunately, this is more common than rare as patients are frequently given a list of things they are to do for treatment consecutively by providers. The physician tells the patient four things he or she needs to do, then the nurse may list an additional three things to do, followed by another list from the pharmacist. It is easy to see how the multiple items can become confused. Planned previewing of information can have the opposite effect by enhancing memory. The effects of advanced organization affirm that previewing information and organizing that information into categories can reveal relationships that can enhance learning (Feldman and McPhee, 2008; Sousa, 2006).

The cognitivism theory does provide some ideation of what may occur mentally in the educational processes of teaching and learning while offering educators some tactical considerations for information construction and delivery (Marr, 1971; Willshaw and Buckingham, 1990). With regard to learning, cognitivists do support the position that detailed, meaningful, clear, organized information is easier to understand, use, and apply (Demetriou and Raftopoulos, 2005; Feldman and McPhee, 2008; Sousa, 2006). Cognitivism also highlights some motivating aspects of learning and retention through identifying the power of meaningful information in learning and the memory creation that occurs with interest or strong emotional ties to content (Demetriou and Raftopoulos, 2005; Feldman and McPhee, 2008; Knowles, 1968, 1972; Ross, 2006; Stuart-Hamilton, 2006). Cognitivism requires the educator to link information to the student. Information linking, according to cognitivism, may occur through the linking of new knowledge to known knowledge, through rehearsal and practice, or through mental connections accessed through emotional ties (Feldman and McPhee, 2008; Sousa, 2006).

Constructionism

Constructionism is a psychological theory of knowledge acquisition that is viewed as a core theory of learning. Constructionism asserts that learners construct knowledge and meaning from their experiences and that each learner individually defines new information using their experience. Constructionists see the mind as a creator of meaning. Constructionism contends that information can be imposed, but understanding is personal and can only come from within (Feldman and McPhee, 2008). This theory posits that the individual learner determines the significance of information through the convergence of self-knowledge and experience with new information (Lund et al., 2005; Saunders, 1992). According to constructionism, without the mental personalization of information, all information presented would simply accumulate in storage in the brain. When information is received, the learner merges new and previous information through mental processing or "construction," yielding a new representation (Lund et al., 2005; Saunders, 1992). The new mental representation, or "construct," incorporates meaning intrinsic to the person. The new construct possesses meaning, which embodies the learned information through a personal understanding. Constructionism captures the individualism of the learned experience inclusive of personal experience, previous knowledge, and the uniqueness of knowing (Bruner, 1990).

Insults in Health have Different Effects on Individuals

Dolly, an occupational therapist at the local hospital, and Kim, a teacher at the local high school, have been diagnosed with breast cancer, and both of their surgeons recommend total mastectomies. As an occupational therapist, Dolly has cared for many patients who have had breast cancer. Dolly is familiar with several of the treatment options available and their success rate. Kim has lost a mother and sister to breast cancer. Neither Kim's mother nor her sister had total mastectomies. Kim was present for all of the treatments her mother and sister went through. Although Dolly and Kim have the same diagnosis, their personal experience and previous knowledge of the diagnosis are very different. Although the information provided about Dolly and Kim is only a snapshot of their different exposure and history to a diagnosis of breast cancer, it helps to display immediate variance in personal influence. The personal influence from life and knowledge will ultimately have bearing on Dolly's and Kim's construction of meaning for their diagnosis.

Penny, the social worker for the hospital, has been assigned to both Dolly's and Kim's cases. After listening to both their histories and their personal exposure to breast cancer, Penny decides in their individual visits to offer both Dolly and Kim her contact information and schedule a follow-up visit with them for next week. Dolly states she does not want to wait because she will be having her surgery next week and would like to know now what she needs to do. Kim, on the other hand, tells Penny that she appreciates her time and she will see her next week at her scheduled appointment. Both patients have the same diagnosis, but both patients are at different points in their processing of the information and decisions to act. Penny allowed both patients the autonomy to freely move at their own pace.

EXPERT SUPPORT FOR ACTION

Fear, lack of control, and grieving for loss of health are all emotions that patients are likely to experience in healthcare (Jervey, 2001; Mitchell et al., 2008). Kübler-Ross identified five stages of grief that are commonly seen in persons who experience loss (Kübler-Ross, 1969). Loss ranging from death to loss of a job can trigger the grief process. The five stages of Kübler-Ross's grief cycle include denial, anger, bargaining, depression, and acceptance. Kübler-Ross described grief as an individual process, whereas Hamilton noted the fluidity and nonlinear nature of the grieving process (Hamilton, 2005; Kübler-Ross and Kessler, 2005). The entire decision process, is influenced by the patient's health status and other influences like physical, mental, financial, environmental, social, culture, and spiritual beliefs (Falvo, 1994; Henderson, 2002; Pierce and Hicks, 200; Prossier et al., 2003; Stewart et al., 2000).

Piaget's work in the identification of the mechanisms used in the process of internalizing knowledge serves as the core for the constructionism theory. According to Piaget, new knowledge is constructed through the processes of accommodation and assimilation (Ausubel et al., 1986; Lund, et al. 2005; Novak, 1998; Saunders, 1992). Accommodation is the process where reframing of the mental representation occurs to accommodate the inclusion of new information (Atherton, 2009). Accommodation is a more advanced process than assimilation, which involves the rearranging of present knowledge (Feldman and McPhee, 2008). In accommodation, previous knowledge is altered to allow for the inclusion of newly acquired information. Accommodation requires learner effort in mental processing, cognitive storage, and practice (Ormrod, 2008).

Conversely, in assimilation, the new information joins into an existing cognitive framework without changing that framework (Ausubel et al., 1986; Lund et al., 2005; Novak, 1998; Saunders, 1992). The assimilation process is relatively passive because the new information is similar and easy to associate with previously embedded information. Although Piaget's work was paramount to constructionism theory, American psychologist Jerome Bruner first introduced the concept of learning as knowledge building or construction (Bruner, 1990; Feldman and McPhee, 2008). Bruner built on the work of Lev Vygotsky, a Soviet psychologist who introduced scaffolding as a method of teaching in education (Ausubel et al., 1986; Feldman and McPhee, 2008; Saunders, 1992). Scaffolding is a method by which the instructor provides support and guidance for a student as he/she transitions to a higher level of thinking or skill (Ausubel et al., 1986; Feldman and McPhee, 2008;

Saunders, 1992; Sthapornnanon et al., 2009). Once the skill is mastered, fading then occurs, which is the gradual removal of support. The student is then poised to successfully function independently (Lipscomb et al., 2004; Sthapornnanon et al., 2009).

Because constructionism highlights the personalization of the learning experience, an active learner is needed for successful learning (Ausubel et al., 1986; Saunders, 1992). Constructionism teaching methods use problem solving, thinking strategies, discussion, and real-world situations to teach learners (Mayer, 1987; Sthapornnanon et al., 2009). Learning heightens in situations that help link information through active knowing and doing (Mayer 1987; Sthapornnanon et al., 2009). These situations may be real world, simulation, or case study. Whatever the context, the learning situation requires the learner to solve problems and build upon existing knowledge. The teacher stimulates thinking by asking questions and offering feedback, but the student is encouraged to resolve the situation via personal conclusions (Meek, 2009; Mayer, 1987; Sthapornnanon et al., 2009).

How Nancy, a Patient Educator, Guided a Patient From a Passive to an Action State in Taking His Blood-Thinning Medication

After teaching Mr. Johnston, the president of the local bank about Coumadin, patient educator Nancy started asking Mr. Johnston how he would respond if he noticed blood in his stool or urine. Nancy did not provide Mr. Johnston with the answer. Instead, she listened as Mr. Johnston walked Nancy through exactly what he would do, step by step. Nancy provided feedback and guidance, but Mr. Johnston had to move the passive information into an action state.

EXPERT SUPPORT FOR ACTION

Redman (2007) asserts that patients need a rationale for ordered treatment, especially when behavioral change is involved. Bloom's original taxonomy moved from the lowest level of thought: knowledge through comprehension, application, analysis, and synthesis, to the highest level: evaluation (Bloom, 1956). As the student moves from knowledge toward evaluation, his or her ability to comprehend and use information becomes more complex. Progression up Bloom's taxonomy follows the student's mental transitioning of information from familiarity to ownership and, finally, to mastery. The capacity to apply logic and be rational in the processing of information exposes more of the higher-level function of the human brain (Ramey, 2005; Roland, 2008). Immediate use of learned information can boost the retention rate up to 90% (Ormrod, 2008; Sousa, 2006).

Two general frameworks described later can be used to create a constructionist learning environment (Feldman and McPhee, 2008). The first framework is Bybee's 5Es—engage, explore, explain, elaborate, and evaluate (Bybee, 1966; Lord, 1997).

1. Engage: find out the extent of student knowledge about a topic, what needs to be known, and then stimulate the student's interest to know more.
2. Explore; allow the student to get involved with the learning materials while sharing what he or she are thinking, observing, and experiencing.
3. Explain: provide opportunity for the student to make sense of his or her discoveries and analysis. Allow the student to identify and interpret while providing correct information as the facilitator of the experience, so the information learned is correct information.
4. Elaborate: allow the student to use understanding of the concepts in new situations, while comparing their previous experiences with their new ones.
5. Evaluate: at every stage of the model, provide feedback and direction, while assuring that correct understanding is being achieved.

The second framework is known as the learning cycle, which has a three-step design.

1. Discovery: the teacher allows the student to generate questions and hypotheses from working with various sources.
2. Concept introduction: the teacher works with the student to help them work through questions, hypotheses, and experimentation designed to stimulate understanding.
3. Concept application: the student moves the problem into new situations in quest of resolution and greater understanding.

In summary, constructionism focuses on strategically building knowledge by gradually adding new knowledge to old knowledge, while incrementally moving the student to a higher level of knowing. The educator focuses on ensuring proper placement of new knowledge so that the appropriate connections are made, resulting in a solid construction. Constructionism helps the educator understand the importance of a discovery and exploration of the safe zone, so the student can sample real-world experiences without real-life consequences. The educator selects projects that can advance the student's knowledge base. A constructionist educator's intent is for the student to safely be able to explore new information under supervision and guidance. The educator serves to facilitate and support the student's mental connections.

Each of the three learning theories reviewed in this chapter: behaviorism, cognitivism, and constructionism, depict the process of learning differently. Figure 5.3 shows each theory and its philosophy toward the learning process. All three theories offer viewpoints that can serve the patient educator as they teach patients. Seeing each patient interaction as an opportunity to add knowledge correlates with the behaviorist view that each pupil's mind in learning is like filling a box. Recognizing the receiver's mind as a computer that processes information, like the cognitivist, helps an educator remember to honor the student's need for time to internally process information. Finally, borrowing the constructionist perspective of knowledge construction can help an educator remember to thoughtfully place information for a solid building of lasting knowledge. Each theory can enhance the art of patient education.

Summary

For learning to occur, information has to have logical order for the brain to receive the information, process the information, and ultimately, to store the information.

Planning and preparing patient information, just as a teacher plans and prepares student information, offers an opportunity for healthcare providers to capitalize on proven academic techniques that can improve the possibility that the receiver, the patient, is successful in understanding the information delivered.

Packaging information for delivery can present a challenge for educators, especially in healthcare.

Many times one-to-one teaching sessions are at the convenience of the educator and do not coincide with optimal timing for the patient.

Scheduled one-to-one teaching sessions can allow the patient to add input to the direction of the teaching interaction. Educators must be open and encourage the patient to identify and share his or her self-diagnosed knowledge needs.

Engaging a learner also involves a physical concerted effort to show the learner that he or she is your present focus.

In constructing and planning what information needs to be delivered, knowing the patient's level of knowledge on a topic is beneficial.

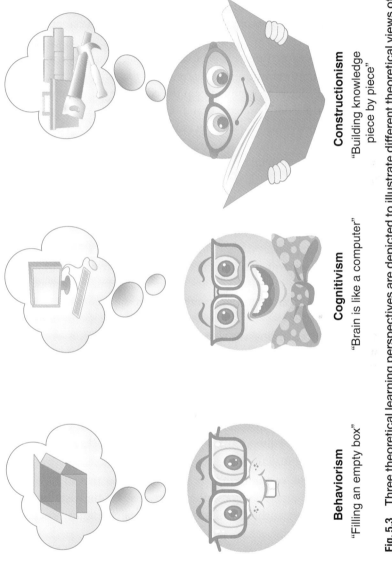

Fig. 5.3 **Three theoretical learning perspectives are depicted to illustrate different theoretical views of learning.** Behaviorism asserts learning is like filling an empty box. Cognitivism views the brain as a computer or processor in learning. Constructionism views knowledge as building or construction, adding a piece of information at a time.

In the 1950s, Benjamin Bloom identified learning domains, which include six levels of human thought that differ in complexity.

Bloom organized his cognitive levels into a taxonomy that many educators use in the construction of educational learning goals and objectives.

In the teaching of patients, understanding the levels of knowledge can help the patient educator in moving the patient from a level of remember to a level of apply.

Teaching and learning are intensely personal activities; not all teachers are the same, and, more importantly, not all learners are the same.

Knowing a person's learning style can help the educator tailor the delivery of information to the learner's preferred (and most effective) learning style.

There are three types of perceptual processing learning styles: visual, tactile, and auditory.

Material delivered according to a personal learning style can help the learner receive and process the information with ease, while increasing the likelihood for overall success in the learner's educational experience.

In learning, knowledge or an understanding is gained by study, instruction, or experience. Learning is a science.

Three prominent theoretical views hold sway in education regarding how learning occurs and the factors that influence learning: behaviorism, cognitivism, and constructionism.

The following theories are considered influences of medagogy:

- Behaviorists define learning as a change in behavior as a result of experience and the creation of habits; they see the mind, metaphorically, as an empty container. Behaviorists believe that human learning can only be explained through observable behaviors.

- Implications for the practice of patient education derived from the behaviorism theory center around the behaviorists' belief that knowledge is not something that exists in the mind, but instead works as a form of guidance formed from actions.

- The cognitivist view of the human brain is similar to that of how the central processing unit in a computer functions. Cognitivists believe that information enters the brain, and then human thought processes the information.

- Cognitivists believe that learning involves mental associations. Humans possess systematic internal capabilities that are used to elucidate their surroundings. Information received is managed according to how it meaningfully corresponds with stored data, called schema.

- Cognitivism also highlights some motivating aspects of learning and retention through identifying the power of meaningful information in learning, and the memory creation that occurs with interest or strong emotional ties to content.

- Constructionism asserts that learners construct knowledge and meaning from their experiences and that each learner individually defines new information using his or her experience. Constructionists see the mind as a creator of meaning.

- Constructionism focuses on strategically building knowledge by gradually adding new knowledge to old knowledge, while incrementally moving the student to a higher level of knowing.

- All three theories offer viewpoints that can serve the patient educator as they teach patients. Each theory can enhance the art of patient education.

CHAPTER 6

Health-Promotion Theories

Because patient education is central to healthcare, it can serve the health-care provider to be aware of existing health-promotion theories. Relate this chapter to one of your themes in Section I that discusses a paradigm shift for prevention, early diagnosis, and intervention. To help the patient educator better understand the relationship that health plays in a patient's acquisition of knowledge, three popular health theories will be reviewed briefly: the health belief model, the precede-proceed health education planning model, and the health-promotion model. These theories offer perspective into three accepted health-promotion theories.

Health Belief Model

In the mid-1950s when public health started to move toward preventive care, a group of researchers at the US Public Health Service developed the health belief model (Green, 2002; Kirscht et al., 1966; Rosenstock, 1966). The model explained and predicted health behaviors stemming from a person's beliefs about the health problem and health behavior. In the mid-1970s, health behaviorist Marshall Becker made some changes to the model by adding measurement scales. For health education, the health belief model remained in vogue as the most used theoretical framework until the early 1990s (Green, 2002).

The model contains four basic elements based on a person's belief of their perceived susceptibility, severity, personal benefit, and cues to action (Davies, 2006; Green, 2002; Rosenstock et al., 1988). If a person feels there is significant personal risk for a health problem, he or she may consider action. If the personal benefit of action outweighs the perceived barriers to action, then action toward change may be considered. If the person feels that they could successfully perform the new action, then action is more likely to occur (Davies, 2006; Green, 2002; Redman, 2001; Rosenstock, 1966; Rosenstock

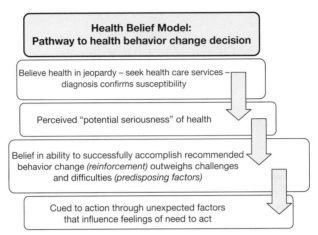

Fig. 6.1 **Health belief model at a glance.** The figure walks through each step of the health belief model. According to the health belief model, the patient starts with seeking healthcare services and ends with personal feelings of the need to act. (Rosenstock, I.M., Strecher, V.J., & Becker, M.H. (1988). Social learning theory and the health belief model. *Health Educator Quarterly*, 15(2), 175–183.)

et al., 1988). Figure 6.1 shows the steps involved in the health belief model ending with the need to act.

The health belief model successfully explores the personal impetus for health behavior of people while providing a unique insight into a patient's focus as they contemplate a change in health behavior. Although the model was developed to predict the adoption or rejection of healthy behavior in people, it has been argued that this model is more successful in understanding the cessation of unhealthy behavior (McIntosh and Kubena, 1996; Rosenstock et al., 1988). The model works off two types of variables: the psychological state of preparedness and the belief that action is needed and will be helpful (Rosenstock, 1966). Becker (1974) asserts that empirical data reveals the impact a healthcare provider's personal involvement can have on gaining patient attention and solidifying patient understanding. Being armed with the relationship between the patient's perceptions using the health belief model and the elements that influence a patient's choice to move toward action can aid healthcare providers as they communicate health information to a patient. Consider the patient who is at risk for diabetes because of family history versus the patient who has diabetes and is suffering from signs and symptoms. In the at-risk state, the patient may not be ready for a change in behavior and because no ill effects are experienced related to diabetes, the belief that behavior is needed may not be as strong as the patient that is experiencing ill effects related to the diagnosis.

How 22-Year-Old Leah Overcame Her Negative Feelings and Became a Positive Participant in Prediabetes Care

Leah is a 22-year-old college student. Since Leah enrolled at the local community college, she has assumed a more sedentary lifestyle inclusive of fast food and sugar consumption. At her annual examination, her healthcare provider, Jana, noted the change in Leah's lifestyle and her strong maternal family history of adult onset diabetes. Leah's weight has consistently increased by 8 to 10 pounds annually. Jana began to discuss her risk of diabetes during the visit. Leah gathered her belongings as her provider spoke, but offered no sign that she was listening and no acknowledgment of reception or understanding. After the visit, Leah's mother asked Leah how her appointment went and without hesitation, she responded "fine." The concept of diabetes had no impact on Leah because she could not relate herself to what the provider was discussing. Because she exhibits no symptoms or complications from diabetes, the diagnosis did not "belong" to her, therefore, it was not of relevance to her life. The significance of a sedentary lifestyle and weight gain did not correlate with a prospective change in health related to diabetes.

The next day, Jana called Leah to give her the results from some laboratory work Leah had drawn on her visit. Jana told Leah that her blood glucose was elevated and she wanted her to have more laboratory work done. Leah told Jana that she had just eaten candy before the blood work was done and that she did not feel it was necessary to have more blood work when the values really weren't that bad. Jana started to tell Leah about the damage that diabetes can cause in the body when she was interrupted by Leah who informed Jana that her mother has diabetes and she knows all about the disease. Jana asked Leah if she would indulge her and come to a free meeting at the hospital at 7 PM. Leah asked why. Jana stated that she felt that Leah may be able to get something out of the meeting while helping others. Leah agreed and showed up for the meeting. Jana facilitated the meeting, which was a support group for diabetic patients' families. Leah was frustrated at first when she found out what the meeting was for, but as she listened to the participants, she began to connect with their messages. Discussions of risks and fears, as well as frustrations, filled the hour; before Leah knew it, Jana was thanking everyone for their participation and reminding them of the scheduled time for the next meeting. After the meeting, Leah approached Jana to find out where she needed to go for her laboratory work.

EXPERT SUPPORT FOR ACTION

Emotions add an even greater challenge to patient learning (Dube et al., 1996; Ong et al., 2000). In adult educator Malcolm Knowles' assumptions (1950), he proposes that as the individual matures into an adult, his or her concept of self changes the manner in which learning is approached. In andragogical methodology, the instructor shifts from the pedagogical source of information to the role of facilitator, an expert resource, who helps guide the learner toward knowledge (Knowles et al., 2005). In andragogy, the learner is self-directed, actively seeking and moving toward knowledge. The employment of various resources and methodologies assists the instructor in guiding the learner toward desired information (Knowles, 1950, 1975).

Precede-Proceed Health Education Planning Model

In 1980, Green and colleagues published the "precede" framework for health education planning. Precede was an acronym for predisposing, reinforcing, and enabling causes in educational diagnosis and evaluation. The model consisted of seven stages to be used in the planning of health education. In 1991, Green and Kreuter, revisited the precede framework and transitioned the model (Figure 6.2) into the more useful precede-proceed health education planning model.

As illustrated in Figure 6.2, the precede acronym stands for predisposing, reinforcing, and enabling constructs in educational diagnosis and evaluation. The "proceed" acronym represents policy, regulatory, and organizational constructs in educational and environmental development. Precede provides

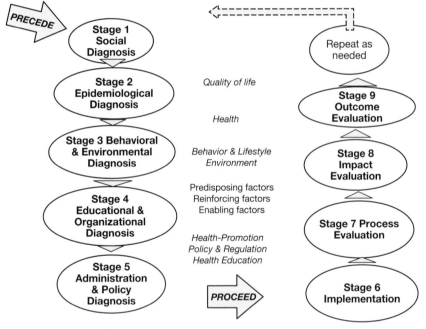

Fig. 6.2　Precede-proceed model. The figure walks through each stage of the precede-proceed model. Precede consists of five stages. Once the user reaches stage five they can stop or transition over to proceed and follow the proceed stages from six through nine. Precede-proceed can be repeated as needed. (Green, L.W., & Kreuter, M.W. (1991). *Health Promotion Planning: An Educational and Environmental Approach* (2nd ed). Palo Alto, CA: Mayfield Publishing.)

a problem-solving strategy to support the planning of intentional specific health-education programs. Proceed complements programs that are designed using precede by providing structured guidance through implementation and evaluation of these programs (Green and Mercer, 2009).

Historically, the precede-proceed model has been used to organize and provide direction for the development of health programs for populations. The model is used to plan and organize activities over time to meet certain health-related goals (Green and Kreuter, 2005). Precede consists of four stages, which are followed by four stages of proceed. The stages of precede are social assessment and situational analysis, epidemiology assessment, educational and ecological assessment, and administrative and policy assessment. Proceed consists of intervention implementation, process evaluation, impact evaluation, and outcome evaluation (Green and Kreuter, 2005). Each of the eight stages has a specific focus for the user to concentrate on as they progress in planning, implementation, and finally, evaluation (Green and Rabinowitz, 2009). The precede-proceed model is intended to flow in an uninterrupted cycle with proceed stages to follow immediately after the precede stages (Green and Mercer, 2009). The stages of precede progress into the stages of proceed as the flow of the model brings the user from broad to detailed in implementation, then detailed to broad in evaluation.

The area of concentration in each stage helps move the user from a universal overarching intent to an action, which is implemented and then evaluated as the user moves back through each stage to the original universal overarching intent. The model covers all aspects by moving from a global concentration down through a narrowing of the focus for intervention then back to the global concentration by expanding the focus as one progresses through evaluation. The flow of precede-proceed offers a logical solid platform on which to build a public health-education program; however, individual education is not the focus of the precede-proceed model. This model is commonly used to strategically plan for community courses related to a specific diagnosis or prevention programs.

Health-Promotion Model

The health-promotion model (HPM) created by Nola Pender was first published in 1982. Pender's model is based on two theories. The first parent theory used to construct Pender's model was from the work of psychologist Albert Bandura, whose social cognitive theory focused on personal self-confidence related to action. Bandura's theory explained human behavior through constant interaction of cognitive, behavioral, and environmental influences (Bandura, 1977). The second theory Pender used, Fishbein's expectancy value theory, is also from the field of psychology. It postulates that people are more likely to participate in an activity they feel is valuable and achievable (Fishbein, 1963). Pender revised her model in 1996 to increase explanatory power and the model's use in creating health-promoting actions (Peterson and Bredow, 2009).

Pender's model strongly supports the partnership between the provider and the healthcare consumer. The HPM serves to provide an understanding of the process people participate in to choose whether they will engage in health-promoting behaviors (Pender et al., 2002). The HPM connects the consumer's individual choices to specific competing preferences and demands to commitment, and finally to behaviors.

Pender et al. (2002) list seven assumptions for the Pender HPM model. These assumptions are:

1. People desire an environment in which they can achieve their unique health potential.
2. A person has the ability for reflective self-awareness and self-assessment of personal competencies.
3. An individual's value grows in a positive direction as they strive to achieve a balance between change and stability.
4. People seek to control their own behavior.
5. People interact with their environment; because of this they are changed, and the environment is changed.
6. Healthcare professionals are a part of the environment and have influence on people throughout their lifespan.
7. Ultimate control is with self; self-initiated alteration of the person-environment relationship is necessary for behavioral change.

There are eleven concepts in Pender's HPM. The first concept, personal factors (biological, psychological, and sociocultural) consists of the factors associated with the person, such as race, physical activity, and family; these factors influence health-promoting activity (Peterson and Bredow, 2009). The next concept, prior related behaviors, refers to an individual's previous exposure to the health-promoting behavior. Behavior-specific cognitions and affect have six concepts: perceived benefits of action, perceived barriers to action, perceived self-efficacy, activity-related affect, interpersonal influences, and situational influences (Pender et al., 2002).

Behavioral outcomes, the final category, has three concepts: immediate competing demands and preferences, commitment to a plan of action, and health-promoting behavior (Pender et al., 2002). Pender's model helps to identify the influences involved in personal movement toward healthy behavior. Understanding the multifaceted nature of people, their interpersonal relationships, and physical environments, as they move toward health, can assist patient educators and healthcare providers in understanding their patients and their individual challenges.

More Significant Theories for Patient Educators

The following theories will be briefly discussed: reasoned action, planned behavior, self-management, self-leadership, self-efficacy, interpersonal relationships, social networking, and transtheoretical theory. Healthcare treatment usually requires a patient to change behavior. Behavioral change theories can offer insight about the concepts, relationships, and influences that occur when a patient is contemplating change.

The theory of reasoned action (TRA), a predictive persuasion theory, was introduced in 1975 by two social psychologists, Ajzen and Fishbein. According to this model, personal beliefs and bias directly influence a person's attitude toward a behavior, which in turn directly impacts his or her behavioral intention and ultimately, his or her actual behavior (Fishbein and Ajzen, 1975). The three main concepts of TRA are behavioral intention (BI), attitudes (A), and subjective norms (SN) (Fishbein and Ajzen, 1975).

TRA maintains that behavioral intention is the sum of personal attitudes and subjective norms: $BI = A + SN$. According to TRA, attitudes are individual beliefs about a behavior, and subjective norms are the beliefs of people in an individual's social environment. TRA suggests that a person's individual and social group's beliefs can ultimately impact their behavior (Fishbein and Ajzen, 1975). This theory highlights not only the role personal value plays in the execution of a behavior, but also the importance of external approval, such as family and peer approval, on behavior (Ajzen and Fishbein,1980). TRA serves to provide a conceptual framework defining links between attitudes, social norms, and individual behavior (Ajzen and Fishbein, 1980).

In 1985, after the TRA theory was included in a relevant study, Ajzen concluded that behavior is not completely voluntary as previously thought in TRA. Ajzen added control beliefs and perceived behavioral beliefs as major variables to the TRA model and named his new model the theory of planned behavior (TPB) (Ajzen, 2006). TPB serves to help in the prediction of deliberate and planned behavior, including actual behavioral control as an influence on a person's behavior.

Social Influence and Personal Management Theories

Interpersonal theory and social networking theory are similar because they focus on the influence other people can have on an individual's actions. Social networking theory proposes that networks of relationships help shape a person, his or her beliefs, and ultimately his or her behavior (Hill and Dunbar, 2002). Interpersonal theory focuses on the social aspect of humans and relationships. It relates how present and past personal interactions shape personal choice and action (Sullivan, 1996). Both of these theories concentrate on the role of social influences in personal behavior. Awareness of these theoretical perspectives can assist patient educators as they try to holistically plan for a patient's educational regimen.

Self-management theory concentrates on empowering a person to control his or her behavior (Redman, 2001). In self-management, the use of self-awareness, personal monitoring of internal cues, and use of external cues for healthy alternative behavior enables a person to take control and manage their personal health-behavior choices. This independence allows a person to progress toward personal health goals.

Self-leadership theory, like self-management theory, also focuses on personal empowerment. In self-leadership, personal empowerment can serve as a motivational construct that establishes opportunity through which persons can raise themselves to a level of improved capabilities and performance (Bandura, 1994).

Bandura's self-efficacy theory (Bandura, 1997) concentrates on a person's self-perceived capabilities to control his or her behavior and circumstances in life (Bandura, 1994).

In the self-efficacy theory, a person's perspective of his or her capabilities influences how the individual views the prospect of success when facing challenges. People with high self-efficacy hold a sense of personal ability to accomplish goals. They embrace difficult situations with a desire to master or conquer. Conversely, people with low self-efficacy are filled with doubt and tend to give up easily when facing challenges. During difficult circumstances, those with high self-efficacy focus on ways to succeed, whereas those with low self-efficacy focus on personal deficits and their lack of ability. In Bandura's theory, personal feelings, positive or negative, about self-ability progress beyond the affective realm into the behavioral realm (Bandura, 1994). Self-efficacy theory postulates that personal feeling regarding self-ability influences self-motivation and ultimately, behavior (Bandura, 1997).

Progress Toward Change Theories

Transtheoretical theory (TTM) focuses on the identification of where a person is in regard to personal decision making and commitment to a behavior-changing action (Prochaska, 2009). TTM is composed of six stages: precontemplation, contemplation, preparation, action, maintenance, and termination (Prochaska and Velicer, 1997; Spring, 2008). Each stage of transtheoretical theory is defined according to its proximity to actual behavioral change (Prochaska, 2009).

Motivational interviewing is a counseling technique often used in health coaching to encourage a person to move through the stages of behavioral change (Miller and Rollnick, 2002). Figure 6.3 depicts the inclusion of these final theories as a patient tries to make healthcare decisions in his or her progression toward behavioral change or action. Understanding the mental progression that must occur to bring about action for behavioral change can help identify how close the person is to implementation of the new behavior. This knowledge can help the patient educator ascertain what information the person will need to know and what skills must be mastered for safety and success.

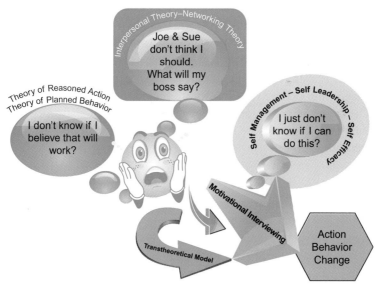

Fig. 6.3 **Patient working toward healthcare choice and action.** The figure shows choice and action theories represented in individual thoughts that might occur in decision-making. The personal thoughts move from considering one's own ability, their social network's opinion, and effectiveness of the proposed action from personal proximity to action. © Melissa N. Stewart.

Summary

- Because patient education is central to healthcare, it can serve the healthcare provider to be aware of existing health-promotion theories.

- The health belief model explained and predicted health behaviors stemming from a person's beliefs about his or her health problem and health behavior.

- The health belief model successfully explores the personal impetus for health behavior of people, while providing a unique insight into the patient's focus as he or she contemplates a change in health behavior.

- In 1980, Green and colleagues published the precede framework for health education planning. Precede is an acronym for predisposing, reinforcing, and enabling causes in educational diagnosis and evaluation. The model consists of seven stages to be used in the planning of health education.

- The proceed acronym represents policy, regulatory, and organizational constructs in educational and environmental development. Precede provides a problem-solving strategy to support the planning of intentional, specific health-education programs. Proceed complements programs that are designed using precede, by providing structured guidance through implementation and evaluation of these programs.

- Pender's health-promotion model (HPM) strongly supports the partner relationship between the healthcare provider and healthcare consumer. The HPM serves to provide an understanding of the process people participate in to choose whether they will engage in health-promoting behaviors.

- According to the theory of reasoned action model, personal beliefs and bias directly influence a person's attitude toward a behavior, which in turn directly impacts the individual's behavioral intention and ultimately, his or her actual behavior.

- Social networking theory proposes that networks of relationships help shape a person, his or her beliefs, and ultimately, his or her behavior.

- The interpersonal theory focuses on the social aspect of humans and relationships.

- In self-management theory, the use of self-awareness, personal monitoring of internal cues, and use of external cues for healthy alternative behavior, enables a person to take control and manage personal health-behavior choices. This independence allows a person to progress toward his or her personal health goals.

- In self-leadership theory, personal empowerment can serve as a motivational construct that establishes opportunity through which people can raise themselves to a level of improved capabilities and performance.
- Bandura's self-efficacy theory concentrates on a person's self-perceived capabilities to control their behavior and circumstances in their life.
- Transtheoretical theory (TTM) focuses on the identification of where a person is in personal decision making and the individual's commitment to a behavior-changing action. TTM is comprised of six stages: precontemplation, contemplation, preparation, action, maintenance, and termination.

Section II Summary

Healthcare practice offers practitioners the challenge of teaching patients who often unwittingly assume the role of student. These healthcare students may be patients or patients' significant others. Most often, the patient does not even realize that he or she are a student and are expected to assimilate all information that is given while a health crisis is transpiring. Too often, the patients and their significant others are so overwhelmed with the emotional component of healthcare that they are unable to sustain the learning component that is inherent to healthcare.

Although academically held principles of teaching can be replicated in healthcare, the student in the patient role is unique and varies greatly from the traditional academic student. Stakes involved with knowledge attainment and learning for the healthcare pupil hold values of life and death in comparison to that of the traditional classroom student, whose greatest risk is having a poor letter grade or course failure. Failure for the healthcare pupil carries consequences such as loss of quality of life, independence, and even death. Information for the healthcare pupil can be life sustaining; therefore, understanding is critical for successful outcomes.

A theory may originate in one discipline; however, the implementation and utilization of the theory is limited only by the beholder. Theory provides definition to concepts with relational statements in a conceptual framework. The value of the theory lies in utilization and application. Theory can be reframed to fit the area of intended application. Theories provide patient educators a foundation of understanding of conceptual relationships while offering a framework for their personal practice in patient education.

Patient Knowledge

CHAPTER 7

Patient Learning

In this section, patient information will be reviewed. Initially, a quick overview will establish focus for the uniqueness of patient learning in healthcare. Then a brief revisiting of shared knowledge from Chapter 1 will transition into an overview of moving the patient from learning to knowing. The following introduction of the author's concepts, evolution of patient information, patient education hierarchy, and informational seasons of patient education serve to add structure to patient education. A brief look at the concepts of medagogy, the art and science of patient education, and measurement of the patient's perceived understanding will conclude this section.

Patient Learning in Healthcare

Aristotle, in the first book of metaphysics, asserted that the main difference between master craftsmen and manual workers lies in the former's grasp of the theory underlying what they do (Aristole, 2009). Aristotle asserted that within the understanding of "why" lies reason, which provides an insight or wisdom that can be used beyond the immediate intended utility. The wisdom Aristotle referred to empowers the master craftsman with the ability to influence beyond original intent to unforeseen possibilities of application, allowing the application of knowledge to be limited only by the beholder of the wisdom.

Healthcare providers, especially nurses, educate patients every day. Patient educators usually borrow individual pieces and parts of facts from various sources with no consistency or personal knowledge of the reliability and effectiveness of the source (Brunetti and Hermes-DeSantis, 2010; Hesse et al., 2005; IOM, 2002). Inconsistency and oversight in the duties of patient education, along with haphazard planning and delivery of patient information are familiar to healthcare (Boyde et al., 2009; Close, 1988). Patients are taught daily in formal planned sessions and through informal, spontaneous interactions. A Swedish study found that, although healthcare providers documented the act of educating patients, the actual patient education was "fragmented and vague" (Friberg et al., 2006, p. 1551). The art and science of the practice of educating patients has consisted of the provider finding the fit, mode, and method of information delivery that tended to work best for the individual provider (Towle and Godolphin, 1999). Often, the act of educating patients is confused with simple exposure to information versus the skillful construction educators undertake so that the information delivered can be understood, processed, remembered, and translated into self-care/self-application (Rogers et al., 2006).

Experts argue that unskilled communication by healthcare providers is to blame for their poor performance in patient education (Hoving et al., 2010; Sandars and Esmail, 2003; Syred, 1981). Schwartzenburg and colleagues assert that healthcare professionals need to be trained in how to teach patients (Schwartzenberg, 2007). Poor patient-provider communication has been linked to a range of negative occurrences in healthcare, from poor health literacy and recidivism to increased hazardous errors (Close, 1988; Sandars and Esmail, 2003). Excuses aside, the multibillion-dollar annual price tag resulting from poor health literacy discussed in Chapter 1 validates the need to move toward definition and organization of patient education among all healthcare disciplines.

Although the profession of academic education provides educational theories and conceptual frameworks that may be used for patient teaching and learning, there are profoundly different learner circumstances that create obstacles on the road to learner understanding when the student is a patient, a receiver of healthcare services (Best, 2001; Gessner, 1989; Kick, 1989). Unfortunately, the learners found in the conceptual models for the educational theories are not equivalent to patient-students; neither are the settings, the stakes, and the messages—basically, nothing but the goal of knowledge transfer is common (Veldtman et al., 2001). The uniqueness of a patient as a student creates the need to look at patient education as a special form of education, separate from traditionally held mainstream education that occurs primarily in academic institutions. Much like the educational awakening that occurred with the founding of andragogy, so is the much-overdue need to differentiate the uniqueness of patient education from traditional education. The medagogy conceptual framework focuses on educating the patient rather than the traditional academic student who is the focus of other educational models.

Healthcare naturally embodies many obstacles for teaching and learning (Behar-Horenstein et al., 2005; Palazzo, 2009). Of course, any environment can pose barriers to learning. When learners must overcome learning barriers, they have increased risk of making inappropriate assumptions that can lead to error (Rogers et al., 2006). In the healthcare setting, learning barriers may be personal, relational, cultural, structural, and societal (Iacono and Campbell, 1997; Spath, 2008; Veldtman et al., 2001). Personal learning barriers can include emotional and cognitive constraints as well as values and belief limitations (Gerteis et al., 1993). Relational learning barriers may include the issues in the history and background of the provider-patient relationship, caregiver-patient relationship, and physical disharmony; these factors may be unspoken, yet communicated through body language (Anderson et al., 2004; Roter, 1977). Cultural barriers may include variance in provider and patient cultures and/or differences in educational background or learning culture (Falvo, 1994; Galanti, 2008; Institute of Medicine of the National Academies, 2009). Structural barriers may include physical setting or teaching-learning environment (Lorig, 1992). Societal barriers reference regulatory mandates, credentialing requirements, and professional standards regarding patient education (Falvo, 1994; Stewart, 2008). In addition, societal barriers contain assumed societal structures differentiating separate roles, classes, rights, and privileges, as well as organizational values and financial constraints or incentives, productivity requirements, and time value or constraints (Galanti, 2008; Roter, 1977; Wlodkowski, 2008).

Moving Toward Shared Knowledge

In the healthcare setting, licensed healthcare providers serve as authorities on health, healthcare, disease, and treatment knowledge content (Roter, 1977; Towle and Godolphin, 1999). The licensed healthcare provider serves as an expert of subject matter (health, healthcare, treatment, and disease). The patient, on the other hand, serves as an expert of self in the patient-provider relationship. The patient is uniquely positioned to possess full understanding of his or her personal life, feelings, and all that has consciously been experienced by self (Brodenheimer et al., 2002; Funnell and Anderson, 2004). Using their expertise, both experts, the patient and the provider, have influence and power that can contribute to finding answers to reach successful health outcomes (Towle and Godolphin, 1999; Wingate, 1990). The key to being successful in the patient education process lies in the success of open, nonjudgmental patient-provider communication (Institute of Medicine of the National Academies, 2009).

Information needs to be openly exchanged in the provider-patient relationship. Information withheld from either party could directly impact potential outcomes. All information exchanged needs to be received and valued. Being received goes beyond simply hearing. Received means the information is actually comprehended and is mentally ingested. Being valued means the

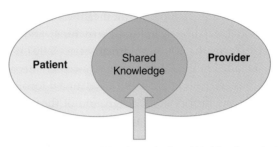

Fig. 7.1 Merging of patient-provider knowledge. Working knowledge is the foundation for partnership on which to plan, care, and build future knowledge.

information has importance and worth. The intent is for both patient and provider to receive and value the information provided and then merge it with personal expertise. The union of new information with personal expertise is used to provide a foundation of understanding that serves as shared knowledge for both parties to use in decision making in the patient-provider encounter (Figure 7.1).

The health decision cycle shown in Figure 7.1 offers a visual of the impact and flow of information exchange between the experts, the expert of health and the expert of self, in the provider-patient relationship. Two conceptual streams are depicted in the health decision cycle: information and choice. The information stream is composed of communicating and listening, which openly flows between provider and patient. Choice also streams openly between provider and patient. Choice and information run alongside each other and then intersect just before the reception of each party's contribution to shared knowledge. Information and choice intersect at both the patient and provider levels, symbolizing the connection or influence each has with the other. The health decision cycle visually displays how information is exchanged between the provider and the patient, while simultaneously, choices emerge between the patient and provider. Figure 7.2 depicts the health decision cycle.

From Learning to Knowing

All men by nature desire knowledge.

ARISTOTLE (384 BC——322 BC)

Trying to learn can be challenging for people, even when they have identified a need for knowledge and are willing and ready to learn. Add to the learning environment the factors that patients may experience like illness, emotions (i.e., fear, anger, insecurity, and sorrow), financial insult, pain,

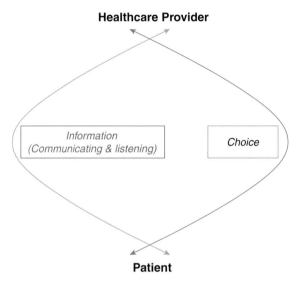

Fig. 7.2 Health decision cycle. The healthcare decision cycle displays a constant flow of information between the provider and the patient. Choice is noted in the display as a constant exchange between the patient and provider. The two constants represented, information and choice, intersect on both the provider and patient ends to symbolize the influence both bear on the other. Choice is influenced by information, and information is influenced by choice. (Green, L.W., & Kreuter, M.W. (1991). Health Promotion Planning: An Educational and Environmental Approach (2nd ed). Palo Alto, CA: Mayfield Publishing.)

chaos, urgency, and more, it is easy to see how learning can become even more challenging (Levinson et al., 2000; Rolls et al., 1994). The emotions mentioned may be encountered but are not traditionally common to student populations in an academic setting, whereas, it is a rarity for these human emotions to be absent in healthcare patients (Clark et al., 2003; Gustafson et al., 2003). It is normal for patients to experience a wide array of emotions while receiving healthcare. Emotions add to the challenge of patient education and patient learning (Dube et al., 1996; Ong et al., 2000). The emotion factor is a unique characteristic common to the patient-pupil.

Fear, lack of control, and grieving for loss of health are all emotions that patients are likely to experience in healthcare (Jervey, 2001; Mitchell et al., 2008). As a patient educator, it is important to recognize and understand Kübler-Ross's five stages of grief that are commonly seen in people who experience loss (Kübler-Ross, 1969). Loss from death, loss of a job, loss of health and/or a normal lifestyle can all trigger the grief process. The five stages of Kübler-Ross's grief cycle include denial, anger, bargaining, depression, and acceptance. Kübler-Ross described grief as an individual process, whereas

Hamilton (2005) noted the fluidity and nonlinear nature of the grieving process (Hamilton, 2005; Kübler-Ross and Kessler, 2005). According to Kübler-Ross, people go through all, some, or none of the stages of grief at their own pace. People may become stuck in a stage or even recycle through a stage more than once. Kübler-Ross recognized that each person is different and that grief is an extremely personal experience with no certainty to emotions or responses in each individual's grieving process.

While trying to educate patients about their health, emotional deterrents may be encountered. Patients in healthcare are vulnerable to experience the stages of grief or loss. Many patients experience loss of control, loss of their (personally defined) health, loss of quality of life, loss of independence, and possibly even loss of self-identity (Penzo and Harvey, 2008; Smart, 2008). Knowing if the patient is grieving or if he or she is experiencing other emotional stress, such as fear, lack of control, or other negative uncomfortable emotions, can help the patient educator as they approach planning and then executing patient teaching. These uncomfortable emotions can be barriers to learning. Therefore, it is important to make accommodations for patients who are, or become, emotionally distraught or overwhelmed by their diagnosis, plan of care, and/or prognosis. Knowledge of these emotional blockades can help patient educators identify when extra resources may be needed. Resources such as a family member or friends may need to be in the patient's informational or educational sessions to assist the patient with his or her health needs as the patient works through their emotional struggles. Careful planning of teaching material and follow-up will be needed to ensure the integrity of the taught material is maintained as the learner mentally ingests and applies new information.

Creating a supportive, respectful environment where a patient feels heard and understood is important to a successful transition through the patient's emotional challenges. Understanding that grief and/or uncomfortable emotions are normal and may surface with any crisis throughout the patient's health management can help the patient educator be sensitive and prepared for each encounter with the patient (Hamilton, 2005; Penzo and Harvey, 2008).

Evolution of Patient Information

The evolution of the patient information model shows the progression of information as it is received and then moves through stages to become part of a patient's knowledge base. The information moves from exposure through instruction to a level of individualization where ownership and control of information occurs. Exposure, the first function in the process of educating a patient, is the most common information delivery seen in healthcare today, and unfortunately, is often mistaken for education. In exposure, information is given to the patient, but preparation of information, delivery, and timing are all based on convenience and provider preference. Information is literally often just handed to the patient in a superficial revealing.

From the exposure level, a more concentrated level of instruction or teaching evolves, moving the communication process toward education in a more patient-centered process. From instruction, information then progresses toward patient ownership, where the patient processes information to include self. The addition of self to the information begins to individualize the information. Clarification and reinforcement, which can be achieved alone or in conjunction with the provider or educator, can help the patient as he or she prioritizes new information and determines the influence that the new information will have on personal choices and behavior. After personal ownership of the information occurs, the patient then uses the information to manipulate the world through choices the patient makes from the new information. Figure 7.3 displays the evolution of information in patient education.

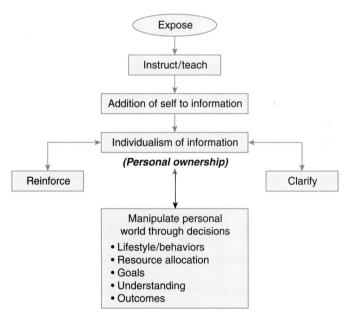

Fig. 7.3 Evolution of information in patient education. The figure displays the progression of information in patient education from exposure to a level of teaching/instruction. From teach/instruct, information can progress to where the recipient inserts self into the information. After the addition, self-information becomes individualized with a need for occasional reinforcement or clarity. After individualism of information occurs, there is personal ownership that empowers the recipient with the ability to manipulate their personal world. © Melissa N. Stewart.

Levels of Knowledge

Knowledge is multifaceted, having various levels to attainment. In academia, educators work hard to move students toward higher levels of knowing. Movement occurs in stages and grades, and not all students learn are at the same pace, resulting in students with various levels of knowledge. As reviewed in Chapter 5, one tool frequently used in academia is Bloom's taxonomy, a nomenclature of levels of human thought (Bloom, 1956). The taxonomy offers educators a guide to use as they target where each student needs to be in their acquaintance with information. The taxonomy assists educators in planning goals for a student's knowledge attainment and progression. Bloom's original taxonomy moved from the lowest level of thought—knowledge through comprehension, application, analysis, and synthesis, to the highest level—evaluation (Bloom, 1956). As the student moves from knowledge toward evaluation, his or her ability to comprehend and use information becomes more complex. The progression up Bloom's taxonomy follows the student's mental transitioning of information from familiarity to ownership and, finally, mastery.

At present in healthcare, mastery is least attained, and mere exposure is the level at which most patient education attempts remain (Moons et al., 2001). This lack of focus on the progression of human thought has many implications; two are readily identified: safety and consent, or informed decision. Patient education calls for a hierarchical approach to establish order to the patient's progression of knowledge attainment. The lack of mastery can have life and death consequences for the patient, versus the traditional classroom student (Osborne, 2005). The hierarchy offers a focus for prioritizing a patient's knowledge needs (see Figure 7.4). As the patient's knowledge migrates up the hierarchy, greater independence and self-determination are realized by the patient.

The foundational level of hierarchy focuses on safety. This level must be achieved and maintained for any higher level of learning to occur. Maintaining safety will help to avoid preventable setbacks in health. Maintaining safety allows the patient and healthcare provider to focus on health and knowledge progression. For example, teaching a patient how to ambulate safely and to make sure pathways are well lit and uncluttered can help prevent falls and related injuries like fractures and sprains. Another example is safe medication administration of alternating Coumadin dosages. Making sure the patient understands how to administer their Coumadin safely can help prevent too much or too little of the ordered dosage. Avoidance of potential safety hazards such as these helps

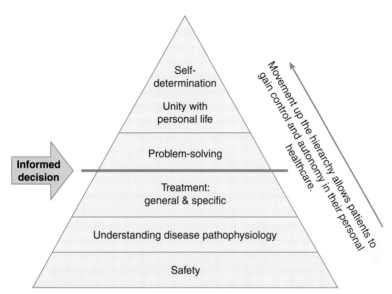

Fig. 7.4   Patient education hierarchy. the hierarchy provides a method to approach patient education prioritization. The foundational level of the hierarchy is safety. It is imperative that the patient always receives safety instruction first, progressing from the foundation up the hierarchy, moving from disease process through treatment to problem solving. The final level represents the culminating point of patient education, self-determination, where the patient is in control of health, inclusive of any disease state. © Melissa N. Stewart.

to maintain the patient's momentum toward improved health, maintains patient confidence, and allows the patient to concentrate on the next level of knowledge on the hierarchy.

The second level of the hierarchy, disease pathophysiology, offers patients an opportunity to understand normal pathophysiology of the body and what is happening in their bodies, chemically and physically, because of their health state. This understanding of physical and chemical circumstances helps to form a justification or rationale for the treatment plan. Having the "why" for the treatment plan helps to ease the patient's knowledge transition into the next level of the hierarchy. The third level, treatment, entails the treatment the patient is expected to follow. Treatment may include a range, from generic, universally used treatment, such as daily weight measurement for congestive heart failure patients, to individual treatment that is patient specific, such as a prescribed heart-healthy diet regimen tailored to accommodate individual allergies.

Multiple reviews may be needed, but once the patient understands the information, he or she now has the knowledge base to actively participate and knowledgeably regulate their care. Knowing the pathophysiology and treatment allows the patient to gain perspective into the healthcare provider's reasoning in the formulation of the treatment plan. A solid understanding of pathophysiology and treatment then moves the patient to a level where he or she should be comfortable making informed decisions regarding care. Obtaining a level of knowledge can empower the patient with enough information to be able to ask questions, request clarification, acknowledge that the provider's conclusion is not congruent with their health state, reason through treatment choices, and most of all, personally advocate for self. This level of knowing moves the patient into a more active role in the healthcare relationship by broadening the patient's span of influence (discussed in Chapter 4).

Once the patient has made an informed decision, then he or she will need to have educational support in mastering the disease and treatment information. In the mastering of disease and treatment, problem solving should be applied to evaluate the patient's ability to react and control predictable and unpredictable variables that could influence the patient's health status. The fourth level, problem solving, truly requires an in-depth understanding of the disease, complication management, and treatment protocol before the next level can be reached.

Once the skill of problem solving has been mastered, then the patient has reached the highest level of the hierarchy. At the highest level, the patient no longer sees the diagnosis separate from self. The patient and his or her health state are one; the diagnosis has merged with the patient's identity. The patient controls the health state just as they do anything else in his or her life. Complete and full mastery of the health state has allowed full understanding and management of the diagnosis to unify with their person. At the pinnacle of the hierarchy, through actualization of self, which is inclusive of the health state, the patient reaches a level of confidence and competence in self-care that transitions him or her to a level of proficiency in knowing how to control and skillfully direct the self through life choices and decisions. In self-actualization, the patient is able to comfortably choose the progression and path for treatment within his or her life.

Today's patients with multiple chronic illnesses may be on various levels of the hierarchy at any given time. For example, a patient with diabetes, congestive heart failure, and stroke may be at the problem-solving level for diabetes, pathophysiology level for congestive heart failure, and only at the safety level for stroke. Dealing with acute situations versus chronic conditions may have some influence as to the patient's various levels of knowledge. The challenge for the healthcare provider is to balance the patients' knowledge progression while maintaining their foundational safety level. Safety should always be first when approaching patient education. Lack of safety can negatively affect healthcare outcomes, levels of independence, and knowledge progression because of shifting focus from mental gain to physical gain. It is important to have physical dexterity and independence, but without a foundation of safety, risk of injury or error can impede and/or set back patient progress, gains, and independence.

Information should be structured so the patient progresses up the hierarchy toward the level where informed decision can be accomplished, and then continues toward the apex of the hierarchy where the patient achieves full control of his or her health status as the knowledge becomes one with self. Once at the top level, self-determination begins as the patient has gained mastery of the health-state knowledge and unifies the health state with self. The patient redefines self, inclusive of all of his or her other knowledge and skills, including knowledge and skill of health. A new self emerges, comprised of health conditions or diagnosis of illness as a part of self just like an arm or leg. No longer is the health state a burden or label, instead, it is part of the person.

Taking Action After Bariatric Surgery Prevents Serious Complications

Janet, a 36-year-old Native American female, works as the town's librarian and has a history of morbid obesity and hypertension. Janet recently elected to undergo bariatric surgery. She has been prepared for her new diet and lifestyle through multiple preoperative visits. Now that Janet has had the surgery, she is in pain and is suffering from extreme bouts of nausea and vomiting. The food she had purchased preoperatively to eat when she returned home from surgery is not settling well with her "new" stomach. Because Janet understands the risk of malnutrition with bariatric surgery, she decides she needs to call her surgeon for direction. Although Janet has reservations about "bothering" her surgeon, she feels the fact that her present state is not improving, and she must do something. Janet's copay for emergency room visits also serves as an impetus for the physician call.

After the call to the surgeon, Janet felt comfortable that she knew what to do to help decrease her nausea and vomiting. Janet's appropriate actions in accessing the healthcare system through her surgeon (primary care for this issue) saved her from suffering a potential negative consequence like dehydration or electrolyte imbalance. Janet's functional understanding of the surgery she underwent and her astuteness in correlating the prospective negative her emesis could ultimately have on her health allowed Janet to act independently and appropriately. Without Janet's early intervention, she may have been hospitalized, costing her more time and money over something that was preventable.

Information from the lower three levels of the hierarchy will always require reinforcement. Reinforcement will help to keep the information fresh and in the forefront of the patient's mind. The number of health conditions and diagnoses, along with personal health information "season" can be a challenge in a person's attainment of hierarchy levels and knowledge progression.

Summary

- Aristotle, in the first book of metaphysics, asserted that the main difference between master craftsmen and manual workers lies in the former's grasp of the theory underlying what they do. Aristotle asserted that within the understanding of "why" lies reason, which provides an insight or wisdom that can be used beyond the immediate intended utility.

- The art and science of the practice of educating patients has consisted of the provider finding the fit, mode, and method of information delivery, which tended to work best for the individual provider.

- Experts argue that unskilled communication by healthcare providers is to blame for their poor performance in patient education. Schwartzenburg et al. (2007) assert that healthcare professionals need to be trained how to teach.

- The uniqueness of a patient as a student creates the need to look at patient education as a special form of education, separate from traditionally held mainstream education that occurs primarily, in academic institutions.

- The licensed healthcare provider serves as an expert of subject matter (health, healthcare, treatment, and disease). The patient, on the other hand, serves as an expert of self in the patient-provider relationship.

- Information needs to be openly exchanged in the provider-patient relationship. Information withheld from either party could directly impact potential outcomes.

- It is normal for patients to experience a wide array of emotions while receiving healthcare. Emotions add an even greater challenge to patient learning. The emotion factor is a unique characteristic common to the patient-pupil.

- Understanding that grief is normal and may surface with any crisis throughout the patient's health management can help the patient educator to be sensitive to each encounter with the patient.

- At present in healthcare, mastery is least attained, and mere exposure is where most patient education attempts remain.
- Knowing the pathophysiology and treatment plan allows the patient to gain perspective into the healthcare provider's reasoning in the formulation of the treatment plan. A solid understanding of pathophysiology and treatment then moves the patient to a level where he or she should be comfortable making informed decisions regarding care.
- This level of knowing moves the patient into a more active role in the health care relationship by broadening the patient's span of influence.
- In self-actualization, the patient is able to comfortably choose the progression and path for treatment within his or her life.

CHAPTER 8

Informational Seasons of Knowledge

Because of the magnitude of influence that information has in the provider-patient relationship, it is important to prepare patient information not solely on the receiver's understanding and retention needs but also according to the impact experienced personally from the health condition. In medagogy, three levels of health impact are used. These levels are referred to as health informational seasons. Informational seasons offer a new way of looking at patient communication and learning. They help the educator to adjust the patient information to be delivered for the position or place the patient is in their health.

Just as all patients are uniquely individual in their different needs, so are the timings of patient healthcare access.

Applying Health Informational Seasons to Hypertension in Three Patients

Michael, the local Boy Scout troop leader, is a hypertensive patient who now requires medication and a low sodium diet. Marlene, the town's local artist, is a hypertensive patient who suffered a stroke secondary to her hypertension. Phyllis is a young mother who works part-time as a cashier at the local market and has a family history of cardiovascular disease but no personal active diagnosis of hypertension. All three individuals are at a very different stage of health. All three patients are also at very different informational seasons in their health even though they share the same actual or potential diagnosis: hypertension.

Given the variance of patients' health seasons, it is important to capture their personal season or timing by presenting information according to the present health position on the continuum of the disease and health. Whether the patient is in the final days of living with a terminal illness, or whether they run the risk of developing a diagnosis because of personal or family history, the patient's information must address their individual health season.

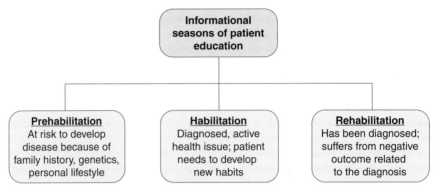

Fig. 8.1   Informational seasons of patient education. The figure displays the three informational seasons of patient education. Prehabilitation is the season before disease onset or injury. Habilitation is the season where active diagnosis is made or a disease state, without the occurrence of deficits or injury, has occurred secondary to the diagnosis. Rehabilitation represents the season where negative insult has occurred because of the diagnosis or health state. © Melissa N. Stewart.

Medagogy identifies three informational seasons of patient education: prehabilitation, habilitation, and rehabilitation (Figure 8.1). Each informational season offers a perspective for patient education construction and delivery to help make information more patient centered while adding personal health-time orientation. Although the same information may be threaded throughout all seasons, the perspective of the patient's position in correlation with the disease and their need to act helps to frame information for that individual patient in their present continuum. Each stage is named according to the patient's relationship to needed personal health-behavior change. The seasons are independent of each other. Transition through one season is not contingent for progression into the next season. A person may transition through one or all of them. It is dependent on the provider's ability to recognize a patient's health status relative to a season and be capable of delivering information that is oriented to the patient's season.

Understanding the Patient's Health Position Enables the Provider to Focus Information

If Michael, Marlene, and Phyllis, mentioned earlier, all shared the same primary care physician and all coincidentally accessed that provider on the same day, the information offered should be centered on where each individual is in their health in relation to the diagnosis of hypertension. Although the same diagnosis of hypertension is the focus of the education, each individual's current health position helps the provider frame the focus of his/her communication.

Season 1: Prehabilitation

Prehabilitation is the season for prevention and promotion through patient education. During this phase, the patient is at risk for or will develop a diagnosis or health condition. The patient may have a strong family history, or their lifestyle may put the patient at jeopardy for developing or contracting a specific illness or health condition. In the case study offered, Phyllis would be in the prehabilitative season for hypertension because of her family history.

For "at risk for" or prevention instruction, this season allows the healthcare provider to appeal to the patient to change their behavior to reduce the odds of onset or risk of exposure. A smoking cessation course is an example of prehabilitation instruction to change behavior as a prevention technique. Prehabilitation instruction could also focus on gaining comfort and mastery of a skill or set of skills in preparation for the health state. A common example of instructing a person in promotion of the prehabilitation season is instruction on protection during intercourse for a nonsexually active person. A Lamaze class for pregnant women is also an example of prehabilitation because of the preparatory instruction for prehealth state onset skill attainment before health insult.

Patients' reactions to prehabilitation education are precarious because the pending health state or diagnosis is not yet a reality. The patient's only life experience with the disease or health condition may be through extension, exposure experienced through social networks, and observation of others. The person may have no experience with the health status and knows nothing about the illness or condition. One such instance could be a pregnant woman who knows no one who has breastfed and knows nothing about breastfeeding. She needs information that she may use after she delivers. The timing of her delivery may influence her motivation. The closer she is to her due date, the more motivated she may be to learn. Distance between the pending health status and the patient may offer a false sense of optimal health to the patient, leaving the patient with a low priority and lack of interest in the information that is being presented in the prehabilitation information season. Lack of urgency may reveal itself in procrastination or denial.

Patient engagement and commitment to action is the greatest challenge for the healthcare provider during the prehabilitation season. Any source of association, risk factors, or reality submersion should be used in relaying the relevance of the information and the need to act. For example, the type of breast cancer your mother had puts you at risk for developing the same breast cancer, or your strong family history of heart disease along with your present weight and sedentary lifestyle put you at a higher level of risk for developing heart disease.

Communicating urgency in the information may spur motivation to learn and act. The link, meaning the reason patients are at risk, must be present to support the prescribed behavior changes to delay or reduce the risk of developing the pending health condition. The "why" offers a solid foundation on which to build a plan of action to address behavior and lifestyle. A patient remains in the prehabilitation season of learning until a change in health status warrants the patient's movement into an active diagnosis or health insult state.

Phase 2: Habilitation

In the second phase, habilitation, the patient has been diagnosed with the disease or health condition. The patient has an active diagnosis or insult to health and may or may not have associated symptoms. In the case study offered, Michael would be in the habilitative season for hypertension because of his active diagnosis and treatment plan requiring an immediate change in diet and medication.

Just like the patient in the prehabilitation season, the patient in the habilitation season needs to understand the "why" of the insult to their health status. In habilitation, the active status of the diagnosis makes the goal of the season to educate the patient in the management or treatment of their health. A solid understanding of the why will allow the patient to better master the management of their health state so they can avoid negative outcomes, exacerbation of symptoms, and further damage due to their health condition.

The patient may not have had any prior instruction related to the health condition and this may be their first exposure to information regarding the diagnosis. If prior knowledge of the disease is present, the next step is for the patient educator to find out what is known. It is important to note that prior knowledge does not mean correct knowledge. Therefore, clarification of misunderstood information is very important and a top priority for the patient educator. If patient education starts without complete clarity of what is known and the assurance that the knowledge is correct, then patient education attempts may lead to chaos and confusion. The patient must possess accurate knowledge.

In the habilitation phase, the patient may be ambivalent about their diagnosis. Lack of any prior history, either personal or familial, and absence of symptoms may only serve to heighten any reservations the patient may have about the diagnosis. The health provider's diagnosis or confirmation of change in the patient's health may act as a catalyst, triggering patient entry into a grieving process. Grief and loss may occur because of the patient's perception of their movement away from optimal health or loss of desired health and well-being (Penzo and Harvey, 2008). The patient may actually grieve the loss of health and/or perceived loss of self. Even the temporary need for healthcare treatment or lifestyle changes may trigger a sense of loss of control and quality of life, initiating the possibility of the patient moving through some, all, or none of the grief cycle. Each stage of grief the patient moves through offers a new challenge to information delivery in the habilitation phase.

The key to success in the habilitation season is to support the patient as they move through emotions associated with an alteration in health and to be prepared when the patient is emotionally ready to move toward a plan. The goal is for the patient's information to be delivered by the healthcare team at a level the patient understands, so the patient is able to use the information. Through work, patience, and acceptance, the patient may be able to move beyond understanding to control and merge information into their life.

Ultimately, the provider should strive to help the patient reach a level where self-determination is influenced by personal disease understanding allowing the diagnosis to become a part of self, no longer viewed by the patient as something extra or different. The secret to reaching self-determination lies in the relationship of the healthcare provider and the independence of the patient. Just as the healthcare provider assumes the role of health expert, likewise, the patient should be viewed as the expert of self. The disease understanding that is shared between the two experts is shared common knowledge on which the patient's treatment is planned between the two experts. This shared knowledge will also serve as a foundation for all future disease knowledge information.

This shared knowledge unites information like disease pathophysiology and treatment from the healthcare provider with the patient's individual information like values and lifestyle. The shared knowledge helps to serve as a foundation for a true partnership between healthcare provider and health consumer or patient. With shared knowledge, both parties must accept and understand each other's perspective and expertise, while offering personal perspectives and desires. Shared knowledge empowers both patient and provider with a voice to offer and discuss opinions, make suggestions, and address any issues that could affect treatment compliance.

The term compliance is too generic and misleading, whereas its counterpart noncompliance bears a pejorative tone (Shea, 2006). Compliance is no longer trying to force the patient into a preestablished optimal disease treatment box. Instead, discussion and planning between experts, the patient and the provider, help in the formulation of a mutual treatment consensus. Compliance no longer represents conformity to one perspective but instead becomes the fulfillment of each individual's responsibility to an agreed treatment strategy. Movement from the planned course is no longer seen as noncompliance or capricious misconduct, but instead is seen as an action made from an informed decision (Shea, 2006). This intelligent noncompliance then flags the experts to review and rethink the treatment plan (Trostle, 1988). Hence, noncompliance is replaced with choice and informed decision.

A patient remains in the habilitation season of learning until their diagnosis or health state is no longer active, resolves, or until negative health outcomes occur. If negative effects occur or health declines where adaptations are needed for regular activities of daily living, then the patient moves into the rehabilitative informational season. An example would be a hypertensive patient who has a stroke with complete left-sided residual impairment. The patient might require training on ambulation, feeding, and basic activities of living skill training; this training is the focus of the rehabilitation season.

Season 3: Rehabilitation

Patient teaching that occurs in the rehabilitation season focuses on empowering patients with knowledge that can help them accommodate functional deficits that have occurred secondary to the development and progression of a disease state. In the case study offered, Marlene is in the rehabilitation season and is learning to accommodate for the physical deficits she acquired related to her stroke.

Grief of loss is an issue the patient educator can expect to encounter in the rehabilitation season just as in the habilitation season. In the rehabilitation season, grieving is focused on the loss of perceived individual normalcy or self-image, changes in the routine of personal life, and fear of death and dying. If the health insult is severe enough, then loss of independence may also be a major issue for not only the patient, but their caregivers and family as well.

This phase can occur during a time of major life crisis as the patient tries to sort through options. It is important that information be direct, factual, and reinforced. If the patient has had an opportunity to progress through the prior seasons of prehabilitation and habilitation, it will help in providing a foundation on which to build new information. If the patient has not had prehabilitation and/or habilitation instruction, then the creation of a solid foundation of what is occurring in the body and the correlation of symptoms or outcomes with pathophysiology is required to provide the "why" for the patient to understand risks, options, and prospective treatment.

If an insult to the brain has occurred, such as a stroke, the patient may not be able to mentally recall any previous instruction received. The goal then becomes to make certain that a foundation of why is redeveloped, so treatment plans can be built. Family is likely to be present and at the patient's side because of negative effects from the condition that have placed the patient in the rehabilitation season. In this season, the education focus is on learning to live with and accommodate for deficits resulting from health status insult. The insult may be temporary, but until full recovery is attained, the focus is on making sure that no further injury occurs because of disease or diagnosis.

Family members can be helpful and can serve as advocates for the patient. The focus of all instruction should remain patient centered, making certain that the patient understands. Caregiver, spouse, or those who will be responsible while the patient is incapacitated and dependent on someone else, must be taught just as if they were the patient. These individuals will also need to understand clearly that, although they are not the patient, they must strive to speak for the patients' preferences and needs. Success in follow-through of treatment relies on patient and caregiver understanding of treatment specifics. Ultimately, the goal is to get the patient as independent as possible, with knowledge of the management of the disease or health status and the self-care that will be needed for an improved quality of life.

Rehabilitation may become so manageable that the patient may move back to the habilitation season where the focus of education is on management and prevention of negative outcomes. Prehabilitation can also be reentered if there is a risk for another health status change or disease because of the primary condition that triggered the negative symptoms or outcomes. The patient may cross over all three of the information seasons depending on their health status or multiple diagnoses. The most important thing is for the patient educator to know what informational season the patient is in, so information can be adjusted to accommodate where the patient is, instead of the patient accommodating the information. Informational seasons of patient education are an integral part of the medagogy framework.

Medagogy

Medagogy acts to provide definition to the process of patient learning by identifying the components of informational exchange in the patient education process. The interpretation of medagogy in patient learning begins in a trusting relationship between healthcare provider and patient. In the provider-patient relationship, the provider serves as the expert of health and the patient serves as the expert of self. Within the position of expert is an assumed level of power which has long been comfortably assumed by the healthcare provider (Shea, 2006). Medagogy asserts that no other person can know more about self than self. Therefore, in the patient-provider relationship, the patient must assume their rightful position as an expert of self.

Information flow is continuous between provider and patient. Information exchanged ranges from exposure to instruction, which may include personal facts and data, to casual lighthearted dialogue. Treatment directions and suggestions should be formatted so that patients can understand the information, make personal informed decisions, and follow through with established health plans.

Information received by the patient and the provider is internalized by the patient and provider. As the internalized information begins to assimilate, an individual interpretation evolves. With the formation of the personal knowledge base, individual interpretation cultivates the information, merging it with the patient's personal world. This merging with their personal world inserts the information into personal everyday living. The resulting individual interpretation then helps to guide personal decisions. Decisions are made from knowledge at the point of decision. An example from the patient perspective is such that if an understanding of health status is present, then an informed health decision can be made. An example from provider perspective includes the presence of an understanding of patient person status affecting the ability to make an informed individualized decision.

The entire decision process is influenced by the patient's health status and other influences like physical, mental, financial, environmental, social, cultural, and spiritual beliefs (Falvo, 1994; Henderson, 2002; Pierce and Hicks, 2008; Prossier et al., 2003; Stewart et al., 2000). Physical phenomena include physical limitations like motor control or ability, vision, hearing, tolerance, and comfort (Stewart et al., 2000). Mental activity influences include learning disabilities, cognitive deficit, and illness or treatment haze where mental clarity is hazy secondary to illness or treatment like recovery from surgery or pain medication usage (Falvo, 1994; Stewart et al., 2000). Financial influences include financial obligations, limitations, and constraints (Greene and Adelman, 2003; Henderson, 2002). Environmental influences are related to the physical environment of the healthcare setting, personal home, work, and social surroundings (Curtis et al., 2000; Falvo, 1994; Gabbay et al., 2000). Social influences include cultural, social networks, community, immediate family, and friends' attitudes, as well as accepted and adopted norms (Kravitz et al., 2002). Spiritual influences include personal, cultural, and faith-based beliefs and values (Falvo, 1994; Greene and Adelman, 2003).

Knowledge Measurement

Historically, standard knowledge measurement traditional to academic settings has not been used in healthcare. Tests and quizzes, and performance-based assessments of knowledge are not common practices in patient education (Falvo, 1994; Lainscak and Keber, 2005; Redman, 2001, 2003). Instead, in patient education a loose qualitative labeling suffices as a knowledge evaluation (Escalante et al., 2004; Freeman and Chambers, 1997). For instance, if a person was exposed to information, the healthcare provider may document "able to verbalize understanding" or "able to repeat back" (Escalante et al., 2004; Freeman and Chambers, 1997). Neither of these examples offers insight as to where the patient is in their knowledge attainment. The first example, "able to verbalize understanding" could possibly even be a brush-off from the patient such as, "Of course, I got it." Whereas, the second example, "able to repeat back" is commonly seen in exotic birds and parrots, which is why parroting is a fitting label for this sort of appraisal. Neither example hits the mark of identifying the patient's status in learning, nor does either example give the healthcare provider the ability to follow a knowledge level which can be built upon.

Certified Patient Educator

The Certified Patient Educator (CPE) is trained in the principles of medagogy and possesses the requisite expertise as a healthcare provider or instructor, while recognizing the patient as the expert of self. The CPE, as an expert patient educator, affords the patient the opportunity to be successful when navigating through the continuum of health information.

Moving Forward

In the 1500s, toward the later years of his life, the Italian artist and architect, Michelangelo Buonarroti stated *Ancora Imparo*, as he referenced his accomplished works. In 1847, Ralph Waldo Emerson, in his book *Poetry and Imagination,* translated the famous architect's words as "I am still learning." The phrase, Ancora Imparo has been interpreted as "I continue to learn" (Bucy, 1981) and "still I am learning" (Man Eoin, 2007). Regardless of the specific phrasing of the interpretation, what is relevant and apropos is the sentiment of being subject to perpetual learning. Whether provider or patient, individual health is a theme of study that requires everyone to assume a role of life-long learner.

As healthcare moves forward, patient education must be included as an essential component of healthcare delivery. Transitioning provider and patient to assume a teaching/learning focus with each and every healthcare interaction will involve direction. The evolution of patient information, patient education hierarchy, informational seasons of patient education, patient knowledge measurement, and the assistance of a Certified Patient Educator are all integral concepts that help construct the framework of medagogy, which serves to provide a conceptual framework for the skill of patient education.

Summary

- In medagogy, three levels of health impact are used. These levels are referred to as health informational seasons. Informational seasons offer a new way of looking at patient communication and learning. They help the educator to adjust the information to be delivered to the patient for the position or place the patient is in regarding their health.

- Medagogy identifies three informational seasons of patient education: prehabilitation, habilitation, and rehabilitation.

- Each stage is named according to the patient's relationship to needed personal health behavior change. The seasons are independent of each other.

- Prehabilitation, the first phase, is the season for prevention and promotion through patient education. During this phase, the patient is at risk for, or will develop a diagnosis or health condition.

- Patients' reactions to prehabilitation education are precarious, because the pending health state or diagnosis is not yet a reality.

- In the second phase, habilitation, the patient has been diagnosed with the disease or health condition. The patient has an active diagnosis or insult to health and may or may not have associated symptoms.

- In habilitation, the active status of the diagnosis makes the goal of the season to educate the patient in the management or treatment of their health.

- The key to success in the habilitation season is to support the patient as they move through emotions associated with an alteration in health, and to be prepared when the patient is emotionally ready to move toward a plan.

- A patient remains in the habilitation season of learning until their diagnosis or health state is no longer active, resolves, or until negative health outcomes occur. Patient teaching that occurs in the third phase, rehabilitation, focuses on empowering patients with knowledge that can help them accommodate functional deficits that have occurred secondary to the development and progression of a disease state. This phase can occur during a time of major life crisis as the patient tries to sort through options. It is important that information be direct, factual, and reinforced.
- Medagogy acts to provide definition to the process of patient learning by identifying the components of informational exchange in the patient education process. The interpretation of medagogy in patient learning begins in a trusting relationship between healthcare provider and patient.
- Information flow is continuous between provider and patient. Information exchanged ranges from exposure to instruction, which may include personal facts and data, to casual lighthearted dialogue. Treatment directions and suggestions should be formatted so that patients can understand the information, make personal informed decisions, and follow through with established health plans.
- The entire decision process is influenced by the patient's health status and other factors like physical, mental, financial, environmental, social, cultural, and spiritual beliefs.
- Historically, standard knowledge measurement that is traditional to academic settings has not been used in healthcare.
- In patient education, a loose qualitative labeling suffices as a knowledge evaluation. The Certified Patient Educator (CPE) is educated in the principles of medagogy and possesses the requisite expertise as healthcare provider or instructor, while recognizing the patient as the expert of self.

CHAPTER 9

The Brain and Memory

This Chapter will focus on creating a language that the entire healthcare team can use to deliver patient education. The chapters will consist of a review of memory followed by emotional links, how educators can capitalize on brain capabilities, and the effect of information flow. The patient education informational delivery model (PITS) will begin movement into concepts of medagogy. PITS offers healthcare providers a pathway for information delivery in patient education. Steps of knowledge will take the reader through the patient's internalization process of information received. A brief look at constructing information for delivery to the patient will lead into the introduction of a new tool designed to measure understanding from the patient's perspective.

Memory

Recall that in section II one of the oldest laws of learning was reviewed, the law of exercise (Thorndike, 1932). The law of exercise is based on the concept that repetition progresses information through the stages of memory. The more a person hears the same information, the greater their chance of mentally filing that information away to be retrieved when needed (Feldman and McPhee, 2008; Ormrod, 2008). A review of how memory works may help patient educators to better understand how they can best maximize a person's memory potential.

To create a memory, three processes must occur (Klein, 2009). First, the occurrence must be deposited as a memory. Next, the memory must be of value to morph with previously stored memories. Lastly, the brain must evoke the memory (Klein, 2009). Human memory is divided into three different stages: immediate, short-term, and long-term. Immediate memory has a duration of 2 seconds or less (Higbee, 2001; Minninger, 1997; Sousa, 2006). Immediate memory occurs when external input is initially stored through sensory impression (Feldman and McPhee, 2008). A variety of generalities may be involved in the memory, such as the color of one's eyes, name, clothing or outfit, laugh, spouse, location of meeting, who was standing beside them, and many more (Higbee, 2001). As the moment of registering passes, details of the impression start to fade, leaving only significant remnants of data (Higbee, 2001; Feldman and McPhee, 2008). Immediate memory is also referenced as sensory memory or working memory. If information that enters into the immediate memory does not have a value or meaning to the receiver, then the information is discarded and forgotten. However, if the data does bear significance, then it will progress to the next level: short-term memory.

Short-term memory has a duration lasting from 30 seconds to 2 days (Higbee, 2001; Minniger, 1997). The universally accepted limit of the capacity for short-term memory is seven items (Cowan, 2001; Feldman and McPhee, 2008; Klein, 2009; MacGregor, 1987). The first study to identify a capacity for short-term memory was Miller's 1956 study, where findings suggested that seven "chunks," plus or minus two, constituted the approximate capacity of the short-term memory (Miller, 1956). Chunks are comprised of information grouped according to personal significance (Miller, 1956). The capacity of the short-term memory remains controversial. At present, an empirically supported range from four to seven chunks is accepted (Chase and Simon, 1973; Cowan, 2001; Miller, 1956). Short-term memory links information for long-term storage together through context and the assignment of meaning to information (Higbee, 2001; Klein, 2009). Short-term memory is an active process. Only through the work of rehearsal or repetition can information be transitioned from short-term memory to long-term memory (Feldman and McPhee, 2008; Klein, 2009).

Once information is in long-term memory, it is divided into two areas of information, declarative and nondeclarative. Long-term memory has infinite capacity and limitless duration (Feldman and McPhee, 2008; Klein, 2009; Sousa, 2006). Declarative or explicit information is further subdivided as episodic or semantic memory. Episodic memory includes memories of events, life history, and personally lived moments in time (Feldman and McPhee, 2008). Episodic memories form, store, and are recalled with little ease with little difficulty. Positive feelings associated with the memory can help strengthen it (Feldman and McPhee, 2008). Semantic or declarative memory is the conglomeration of facts and data not related to any event. Declarative memory is the memory most associated with school and learning. Declarative memories are "easy come, easy go." To strengthen declarative memory, it is required that a person work through rehearsal, repetition, or use of mnemonics. (Feldman and McPhee, 2008). Non-declarative memory, or implicit memory, is comprised of procedural information. Nondeclarative memory is the "how-to" memory that is used in the attainment of procedural skill sets (Feldman and McPhee, 2008). Nondeclarative memory is used in the preparation of all licensed healthcare providers and is used every day in the execution of healthcare duties. Nondeclarative memories include skills like irrigating a suction tube, starting an intravenous line, or conducting an interview. Nondeclarative memories are hard to form and are learned through conditioning and reinforcement, but will last for years (Bauer, 1996; Feldman and McPhee, 2008). Practice can make memories. Retention of information can occur through rote rehearsal, practice, and repetition (Higbee, 2001). A specific sequence of information repeatedly revisited can help make connections with already present or stored information (Feldman and McPhee, 2008; MacGregor, 1987; Minninger, 1997). The repeated information reinforces meaning whereas present connections guide new information in learning and, of course, memory.

Emotional Links

Plato once said, "All learning has an emotional base" (Feldman and McPhee, 2008). A learner brings to the learning experience beliefs, values, and interest, all of which have personal significance attached to them. Emotional centers of the brain are interwoven with the cognitive learning areas of the brain (Zins et al., 2004). Meaning is linked to emotion (Feldman and McPhee, 2008). Emotions can affect learning in two ways: through personal emotional learning climate, and memories from information taught. Personal emotional climate refers to the mood of the learner, while he or she is ingesting and processing information (Jensen, 2000). A positive emotional state, especially about learning, can aid in the learning process (Feldman and McPhee, 2008). A comfortable learning environment can help the learner relax, which can facilitate learning and enhance memory (Jensen, 2000; Sousa, 2006).

Memories evoked may stimulate emotions through the memory's connections. The term "*flashbulb memories*," coined by Brown and Kulik (1977), are vivid memories of circumstances under which someone first learns of shocking, momentous, emotionally charged information. The information is stored once but remembered for a lifetime (Jensen, 2000). Flashbulb memories are very reliable memories and are often associated with events like 9/11, the Oklahoma bombing, the Trade Center attack, and the death of prominent people like Princess Diana, Martin Luther King, and President Kennedy.

The relationship between instructor and student can also stimulate emotions, which can affect learning. Emotions can serve as reinforcement or a barrier, and understanding and mastering their use can help the educator in relaying information that can be remembered. As mentioned previously, positive memories can enhance learning whereas negative memories can also seal memories through the emotional charge (Jensen, 2000; Klein, 2009). The likelihood and the accuracy of memories stored in a negatively charged emotional climate are influenced by the personal relationship to the news (Klein, 2009).

Learning alters the brain. The brain physically changes for memory storage. Permanent memories are formed when the same stimulus repeatedly causes a network of neurons to fire together (Klein, 2009; Zull, 2006). Increased neuron signaling generates the growth of more neural branches, increases the density of the area, and stimulates more synapses (Zull, 2006). Repeated firing of a neural network eventually results in the ability to stimulate one neuron in the network, which will cause the firing of the entire network; this in turn will trigger the recall of the associated memory (Zull, 2006). This process helps to prevent cluttering of useless information in the long-term memory (Zull, 2006). When memories are made, the neural forest actually moves, morphing as new information joins with already present information (Zull, 2006).

The goal of patient educators should be to move information regarding diagnosis or health status from immediate memory through short-term memory into the patient's long-term memory. An understanding of the stages of memory in the brain as well as how to assist the patient in the reception, processing, and storage of information in the learning process should be a part of a patient educator's repertoire of knowledge. Knowing how the brain makes memories can help the patient educator establish an environment conducive to learning. The role of disease and/or insult in the patient can cause a deficit in the functioning of cognitive areas which can also affect patient learning. Knowledge of cognitive operational functioning during learning and memory construction can aid the patient educator in planning instruction while taking into consideration cognitive limitations resulting from disease or insult.

Long-term memory serves as a reservoir for personal knowledge. Speed and accuracy of memory retrieval is contingent on both encoding and attributes of the memory (Ormrod, 2008). Memory attributes may ascribe affective (emotional) or contextual (circumstantial) phenomena encountered during the memory event (Albon, 2008; Ormrod, 2008). Retrieval of stored memories occurs through free or cued recall (Albon, 2008; Eddy, 2007; Zins et al., 2004). Free recall in memory transpires without cues (Eddy, 2007), whereas cued recall occurs in response to reminders of the memory (Albon, 2008; Ormrod, 2008).

Once information has been encoded into long-term memory, the objective is for a person to recall the stored information for personal use. Unfortunately, decay, a process where psychologists assume that memories fade, may conflict with the notion of the long-term capacity of memory to hold lifetime memories. Psychologists believe that mostly intricate details of memories fade in the decaying process (Ormrod, 2008). Ormrod (2008) asserts that some memories may simply be misfiled, whereas unused memories may get lost and become less accessible. Educators can assist in memory retrieval by providing clues and hints or details surrounding the memory event (Ormrod, 2008; Sousa, 2006). Retrieving memories is important for patient educators so they can know what a patient knows. New knowledge construction needs to be built on a reliable foundation of understanding (Redman, 2001).

Capitalizing on Brain Capabilities

Education designed to capitalize on brain processes and capabilities is referred to as "teaching to the brain." These techniques focus on methods that will help the learner in receiving, processing, filing, and recalling information. Teaching with brain processing and cognitive storage in mind makes sense, especially in healthcare where time is limited and understanding and application of suggested treatment is critical. Unlike grade school, healthcare providers do not have one hour a day, 160 days a year, to progress a patient toward understanding their health. Therefore, every interaction with the patient must include health information that the patient will be able to understand, retain, and use. Framing of teaching efforts to maximize the brain's ability to understand and process information for storage and personal retrieval helps to alleviate possible errors in information coding and transfer (Higbee, 2001; Jensen, 2000).

One technique of teaching to the brain is based on the fact that people learn information they have previously been exposed to faster than information to which they have never been exposed (Feldman and McPhee, 2008; Jensen, 2000; Klein, 2009; Ormrod, 2008). Before initiating patient teaching, first ask the patient what they know about the information or topic you are about to discuss. Listen for two things in their response: does the patient have a foundational understanding of what they need to know, and is the understanding correct enough that new information can be added?

Does 67-Year-Old Haddie Understand Her Congestive Heart Failure?

Haddie is a retired dietary worker who is 67 years old, widowed, lives alone, and has been diagnosed with congestive heart failure (CHF) for ten years. On evaluation of Haddie's presented understanding of her health status, specifically CHF, she verbalizes as she places her hand to her chest that her "congestive heart failure" (which she says correctly) involves her heart. Haddie goes on to say that to help her heart she takes a fluid pill every evening which makes her get up two to three times a night to go to the bathroom. When asked, "anything else?," Haddie says, "nope, that's all, if I take my pill I can breathe, if not, then I can't." Figure 9.1 represents Haddie's thought processes while she was talking about her fluid pill.

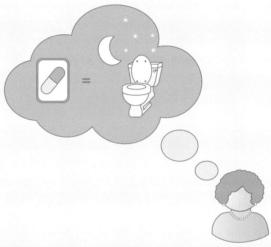

Fig. 9.1 Haddie's mental representation. The figure displays Haddie's thoughts related to her fluid pill and what happens when she takes her pill.

In this case study, the patient, Haddie, is able to correlate the relationship between the medication and the control of disease symptomology, breathlessness, as well as the relationship between the pill and frequent use of the bathroom at night. Overall, Haddie shares minimal knowledge for someone who has lived with CHF for 10 years, but what Haddie relates does provide some insight into her personal understanding of the disease and her treatment. The information offered is correct. Figure 9.2 represents the healthcare provider's thought processes while Haddie was telling her about her fluid pill.

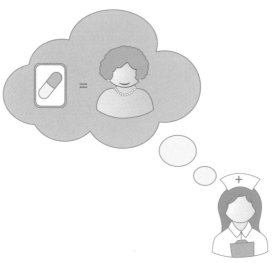

Fig. 9.2 Provider's mental representation. The figure displays the nurse's thoughts of Haddie's fluid pill regimen and it's relationship to a happy, healthy Haddie.

If the information is erroneous in any way, such as if Haddie misunderstood CHF to mean any of the following:

- Diagnosis involving her bladder; believing this is why she urinates frequently at night.
- Normal with seasonal changes; believing her cold medication listing congestion is related to her CHF.

Alternatively, Haddie may have misunderstood her medication (fluid pill) information if she had indicated by the following:

- Her pill is only needed when she is breathless.
- Her pill will heal her heart.

Any misunderstanding of health status or treatment must be addressed before more information is added. The patient educator needs to connect the patient's perception to correct understanding, so the patient, the educator, and the team of healthcare providers share complementary understanding of the patient's health. Time and effort must be invested in using the information that is known, clarifying any misperceptions and making certain that the resulting understanding is correct and usable. Any additional knowledge

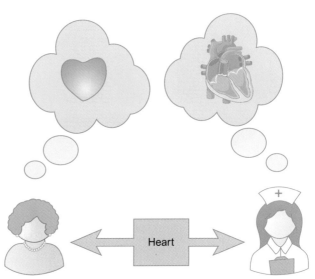

Fig. 9.3   Initial thoughts of heart. The figure displays the two separate thoughts of the patient and the nurse when they think of the heart. The patient thinks of the heart as a pretty valentine; however, the provider visualizes an anatomically correct heart and its functionality.

building will have to be suspended until corrections and clarifications are made and understood. This may appear to be a step backwards to some providers, but this period of clarification and correction should be viewed instead as partnering with the patient through investing personal knowledge and insight in the patient's health. Figure 9.3 represents the initial thoughts of the patient and the educator or provider when the term "heart" is spoken. The figure displays the patient's thought as an average lay person image of a heart, like a valentine heart, whereas the patient educator thinks of an anatomically correct working heart. In Figure 9.4, the thoughts merge because of shared knowledge between the provider/patient educator and the patient.

In another example of reconstructing prior knowledge, Julie, a 21-year-old single female who is 6 months pregnant with her first child, has chosen not to attend any of the free prenatal and Lamaze classes offered. Julie states that she is familiar with labor and the pain of contractions even though this is her first pregnancy. Julie states that she knows that a breathing technique can completely alleviate the pain because her sister Joyce has had three children naturally with no drugs. Julie asserts that if it worked for Joyce, then it will work for her.

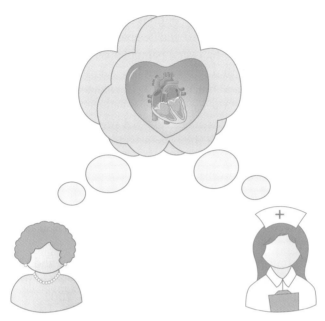

Fig. 9.4 Shared knowledge of the heart. The figure displayed shows merging of the two independent perspectives to create shared knowledge. With shared knowledge the patient has an understanding of the provider's knowledge of the heart and the provider has an understanding of the patient's knowledge of the heart.

Many challenges are present for the patient educator in Julie's scenario. First, correcting the misunderstanding that pain is removed through a breathing technique needs to be addressed. Although the labor pain may be controlled somewhat, complete alleviation is not realistic. When addressing the patient's understanding of contractions, the patient educator should respect Julie's value of her sister's experience while preparing Julie with what physical changes occur in the body during a contraction and how other women have described how the contraction felt. Exposing the patient to what physically occurs in a laboring woman's body will help to provide a factual understanding of what is actually happening during a contraction cycle. Understanding what is occurring in the body allows the patient access into information used by the health expert—the healthcare provider (Boren et al., 2009). Information about the body's physical and chemical processes permits the patient to gain insight into the knowledge that drives healthcare providers' decisions (Williams et al., 2007). Understanding "why" helps to establish a foundational rationale which can be an asset in treatment decisions, for both the provider and the patient (Tokarz, 2009). When the patient then needs to make decisions regarding treatment options that have been offered, they have been exposed to rationale which should be able to support the choices made.

Simply smiling and handing over a pamphlet cannot prepare a patient for an active role in their healthcare treatment like one-on-one instruction of the body's physical and chemical functions can (Hernandez et al., 2009). This instruction helps to heighten the patient's awareness as to where they are on the health continuum (Hernandez et al., 2009). A provider's expertise of healthcare can serve as a resource for the patient with regard to information about which they may have questions. Access to meet a patient's informational needs should be made available to the patient. Once a patient makes an informed decision and is secure in his or her choice, that patient should be supported in his or her choice, free of judgment or criticism. Debating a personal or professional position is not of any value after a decision has been made and should be discouraged.

When educating patients, avoid negative terminology and remarks such as "cannot" or "does not"; this will help the patient's brain in the mental processing of the information (Calvin, 1995; Given, 2002; Sousa, 2006). When negative statements, like "cannot" or "does not" are processed mentally upon receipt, the information must then be reverted to positive, can or does, before the negative can be added and understood (Calvin, 1995). After the information is transitioned twice, the information can be stored (Calvin, 1995). With negative terminology, the process includes receiving the negative information, reversing the information to positive, reversing information back to the negative information again, and finally, storing the information. The extra steps involved in processing negative statements increase the odds of the patient misfiling of the information, which heightens the odds of misunderstanding the information.

How can negatives be taught? By first creating the positive flow of thought and then adding the negative thought after the positive is filed. By first initiating positive thoughts like "can" and "does." then adding the negative of "not," the brain only has to add the negative without having to switch the information independently. Another approach to avoiding negatives is the use of terminology such as, "to avoid this or to prevent that from happening." Finally, an example can be made by allowing the relationship of negative to be imposed by self-discovery, such as with dieting education. Examples such as "calorie intake is important," "for weight loss a 1200-calorie diet is recommended," "anything over 1200 calories will be stored as fat," and "fat stored will increase weight," provide understanding so the negatives can be assumed or self-discovered by the receiver.

The second thing to listen for when evaluating the patient's present-ing knowledge involves patient understanding of what is physically or chemically happening in the body (Boren et al., 2007; Williams et al., 2007). The expectation of a textbook understanding is not realistic, but a rough depiction of what is happening can serve the educator well in ef-forts to progress the patient's knowledge (Redman, 2007). When a build-ing is being constructed, there is a logical order or sequence (Greenburg, 1991; Ormrod, 2008; Redman, 2007; Sousa, 2006). Builders know when they need to hang the front door on a house. The front door is not hung before the foundation, before the walls, and especially, not before the doorframe. For solid quality construction, there is a time for every stage of construction and for every part of the house. The same is true with patient education. There is a time and a stage for every piece of informa-tion if we want to have a solid understanding that can serve throughout a lifetime of health. A solid foundational understanding will allow a lifetime of knowledge construction to occur. Additions and renovations may be needed, but the builder knows the plans and a solid structure will be able to handle it.

Summary

- The law of exercise is based on the concept that repetition of informa-tion progresses that information through the stages of memory. The more a person hears the same information, the greater the chance they have of mentally filing that information away to be retrieved when needed. A review of how memory works may help patient educators to better understand how they can best maximize a person's memory potential.
- Short-term memory has a duration lasting from 30 seconds to 2 days.
- Short-term memory links information for long-term storage together through context and the assignment of meaning to information. Short-term memory is an active process. Only through the work of rehearsal or repetition, can information be transitioned from short-term memory to long-term memory.
- Practice can make memories. Retention of information can occur through rote rehearsal, practice, and repetition. A specific sequence of information repeatedly revisited can help make connections with already present or stored information.

- Repeated information reinforces meaning, whereas present connections guide new information in learning and, of course, memory.
- Memories evoked may stimulate emotions through the memory's connections.
- Positive memories can enhance learning whereas negative memories can seal memories through the emotional charge. The likelihood and the accuracy of memories stored in a negatively charged emotional climate are influenced by the personal relationship to the news.
- The goal of patient educators should be to move information regarding diagnosis or health status from immediate memory through short-term memory into the patient's long-term memory. Knowing how the brain makes memories can help the patient educator to establish an environment conducive to learning.
- Once information has been encoded into long-term memory, the objective is for a person to recall the stored information for personal use.
- Education designed to capitalize on brain processes and capabilities is referred to as "teaching to the brain." These techniques focus on methods that will help the learner in receiving, processing, filing, and recalling information.
- One technique of teaching to the brain is based on the fact that people learn information to which they have previously been exposed faster than information to which they have never before been exposed.
- Any misunderstanding of health status or treatment must be addressed before more information is added. The patient educator needs to connect the patient's perception to correct understanding so the patient, the educator, and the team of healthcare providers share a complementary understanding of the patient's health.
- Simply smiling and handing over a pamphlet cannot prepare a patient for an active role in their healthcare treatment compared with one-on-one instruction of the body's physical and chemical functions.
- A provider's expertise of healthcare can serve as a resource for the patient on information about which they may have questions. Access to meet the patient's informational needs should be made available.
- There is a time and a stage for every piece of information if we want to have a solid understanding that can serve throughout a lifetime of health. A solid foundational understanding will allow a lifetime of knowledge construction to occur.

Section III Summary

When is the last time you heard a lay person say, "Well I'm off to the hospital to learn"? When the general public reflects on healthcare, they think of finding answers to issues they are dealing with while in an environment where people take care of them. Providers reference patient educational efforts commonly as instructions whereas patients frequently reference providers' teaching efforts as being told what to do. When a lay person thinks of education and learning, academic schools are what come to mind, not healthcare. Evidence however, has shown that for optimal health outcomes to be achieved, patients need to learn while they are receiving and/or following healthcare treatment. Health prevention and maintenance cannot occur intentionally without a knowledgeable patient. The new era of value-based healthcare purchasing and patient health assessments such as the Hospital Consumer Assessment of Healthcare Providers Systems (HCAHPS) will demand a knowledgeable patient.

Providers of healthcare bring a wealth of knowledge related to the human body and actions that may impact health and the patient-provider relationship. It is important that the provider is able to effectively assist the patient in gaining understanding of their health status and treatment choices. Recognition that learning is an individualized process and that patients bring unique circumstances to the educational experience can help establish realistic informational exchange. As patients navigate the healthcare system, each provider and access point offer new opportunities for learning. Skill in the teaching and learning process can aid providers as they communicate vital information to patients. As patients master information regarding their health, they can increase their health autonomy and progress to a point where self-determination can be attained. Knowledge of health status coupled with self-expertise empowers the patient as he or she moves toward optimal health.

The health informational seasons of medagogy serve to help educators orient health information in relation to patient proximity to health status and health consequences. The prehabilitation season is where a person is at risk for health implications, whereas in the habilitation season the patient has a diagnosis of an alteration in health status but has suffered no residual insult. The season of rehabilitation distinguishes a phase where the patient has endured a health insult that has lingering consequences secondary to the altered health status. The entry and movement of patients throughout the health informational seasons are not predictive or sequential.

No matter where a person is in their health, they deserve to have information from their healthcare providers that they can understand, remember, and use. Patient teaching needs to be clear and purposeful. Patient educators can facilitate movement of information from immediate memory, through short-term memory, and into long-term memory. Teaching about how the brain learns can help facilitate learning as patients receive, process, file, and recall information. Ensuring that information delivered is encoded correctly can help the receiver properly file data stored in the brain. Information can be accessed more easily when it is filed appropriately. To ensure a solid foundation of understanding, incorrect or misunderstood information should be corrected before new information is added. Patient learning can be facilitated by making sure that information is effectively distributed for successful comprehension.

Information Delivery Methodology

CHAPTER 10

The PITS Model

Information needs to have a logical flow so that it can be easily received, filed, and retrieved. When behavior modification is hoped for, then providing a "why" up front for the desired behavior change can ease the discomfort of confusion associated with lack of access to, and therefore, lack of understanding of the full picture (Jensen, 2000; Redman, 2007). To assist with recall, information should be presented in an organized and logical format (Given, 2002; Slavin, 1995; Sousa, 2006). Information delivered in an orderly fashion makes sense and allows the receiver to easily follow the educator's train of thought (Slavin, 1995; Sousa, 2006). Information composed of pieces and parts that are randomly distributed forces the receiver to assume the tasks of assimilating and organizing the information so it can be mentally filed. Leaving the charge of arranging the order of information completely to the receiver leaves room for error, misfiling, and misunderstanding (Given, 2002; Greenburg, 1991; Redman, 2007).

The organization of information into categories can enhance learning (Feldman and McPhee, 2008; Sousa, 2006). Adding logical order to information for patients does not have to be difficult. Redman (2007) points out that information needs to be delivered in an orderly, sequential style according to the patient's order of need. The author suggests information flow either from disease toward the patient or away from the patient toward the disease. The direction of information may be contingent on the emotional state of the patient or on time constraints. For example, consent for emergency surgery may require information to flow from disease toward patient. The surgeon starts with an explanation of what is happening in the body, what treatment options are available, life implications authenticity, and that consent is needed if surgery is to happen now. Whereas a person having an acute crisis, such as an asthma attack, may need information to flow from patient toward disease. That is, start with treatments the patient needs now and work back toward how the treatment will affect the internal functioning of the body, namely the disease.

Patient Education Informational Delivery Model: PITS

The PITS model was created by the author in an attempt to bring order to patient educational efforts. Order makes a significant difference in the processing and understanding of the information being communicated (Greenburg, 1991; Ormrod, 2008). The PITS model offers a logical organized format to deliver health or disease state information, resulting in a standard communication methodology for the delivery of patient education. PITS in a natural state flows from disease state toward patient; however, PITS can be inverted to change the flow of information from the patient toward the disease state. An overview of material to be covered should be provided before giving new information. This can help let the receiver know what to expect as the information is presented. Knowing where you are going in an educational session can put the learner at ease (Feldman and McPhee, 2008). Delivering the message in pieces will assist in remembering because it allows the mental filing of information into related groups or categories (Greenburg, 1991; Ormrod, 2008).

PITS is an acronym that serves as a patient education model, a common map or pathway for patient education. The acronym stands for pathophysiology, indications, treatment, and specifics. The *P* denotes pathophysiology. Pathology includes all that is physical. The pathology is the segment of education in which the educator identifies any physical changes that have or could occur as the result of a disease, condition, insult, or health state. Physiology refers to biochemical or mechanical changes that occur in the body because of the pathology of disease or insult. The physiology is the segment of education in which the educator identifies any chemical changes that have or will occur because of or in relation to the insult or disease process. During this stage, a patient learns what is normal and what is abnormal physically as well as chemically because of the alteration in health, which the provider deduces from their assessment.

As covered in Section I, Knowles asserts that adult learners need to understand why. Pathophysiology offers the rationale for treatment. Healthcare treatment is ordered to control, prevent, or treat health conditions. Health conditions all have a suspected pathophysiological process for which the healthcare provider formulates actions with which to maximize health based on their knowledge of the suspected pathophysiology that is present. Usually, the patient does not have great depth of knowledge regarding the pathophysiology of the health condition which limits their scope of understanding, further limiting their ability to value treatment options beyond the relationship with the provider.

Has the arguable paternalism of healthcare been the result of provider control or as a result of the lack of the patient understanding the "why" of the health status and therefore the value of treatment recommendations? A healthcare provider's prescribed recommendations are made based on the healthcare provider's expert knowledge of the human body as well as a thorough understanding of normal and abnormal functions of the human body. From the patient's personal report, physical assessment, and diagnostic evaluations, a healthcare provider gathers insight into the patient's health status. Educated decisions are made by the healthcare provider from this compilation of data. Empirical data, standards of care, and intuition are all part of guiding the provider in their decision-making process, but ultimately the pathophysiology is the axis of the treatment decisions. Therefore, allowing the patient access to the axis of treatment decisions may assist the patient in their health choices, which will directly impact treatment outcomes.

Understanding of the pathophysiology also helps establish the association or link between the pathophysiology and the symptomology or indications of the health status. Section II reviewed connectionism and stimulus-response (S-R). Pathophysiology serves as the stimulus for health status indications. Figure 10.1 shows S-R in health teaching.

The *I* in PITS represents indications. Indications are the signs or symptoms that may occur as the result of the disease or health state. Symptoms include what the patient may experience as well as what may be observed or found on assessment. These symptoms may be used as an indicator of disease progression, maintenance, and exacerbation. During the I step, an explanation of indications occurs. The educator should start by reviewing the previously covered material from the P-step, pathophysiology, which includes physical and chemical changes that have occurred as a result of the disease state. Correlating the physical or chemical body changes with the symptoms they may produce or have produced can help the patient better relate to their health status and set the foundation for treatment choices. By teaching the pathophysiology, followed by an explanation of indications, the educator is progressively building patient knowledge in blocks of information. Each block of information adds to and builds on the previous block. The pathophysiology should serve as the stimulus for the response that occurs in indications as seen in Figure 10.2.

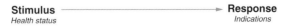

Fig. 10.1 Stimulus-response in health teaching. The figure illustrates the relationship between the health state and the indication to the stimulus-response model.

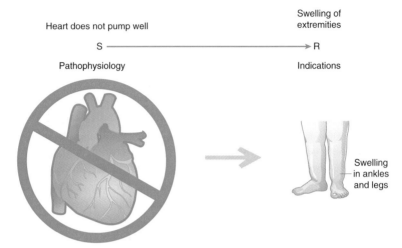

Fig. 10.2 Stimulus-response of pathophysiology to indications of congestive heart failure. The figure illustrates the relationship of the pathophysiology and indications to the stimulus-response model.

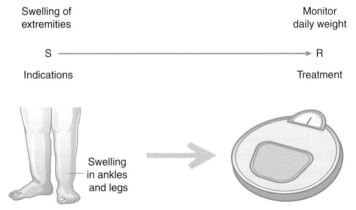

Fig. 10.3 Stimulus-response of transition from indications to treatment of congestive heart failure (CHF). The figure depicts the relationship of the indications and treatment to the stimulus-response model specifically for CHF.

Once P and I are covered, the patient should then have an initial understanding of the provider's view, which directly influences provider decisions in treatment course choices. Redman (2007) asserts that patients need a rationale for ordered treatment, especially when behavior change is involved. The PI of PITS serves as the rationale for the reason a treatment is ordered. Figure 10.3 represents the S-R relationship of the indications and treatment stages of the PITS model.

The *T* of PITS refers to treatment. Treatment is the gold standard or industry-accepted treatment of the disease or health state for which the provider is treating the patient. In this stage, treatment information specific to the disease or health state is provided. Complex instructions need to be broken down and taught one step at a time. This may be information such as how to administer insulin for insulin dependent diabetics or daily weight monitoring for congestive heart failure patients. Pamphlets, handouts, videos, and other educational tools that are available can be used for this stage because the information is not specific to the patient. Just like the previous step, in the T step, it is useful to go back and build on the information covered in the P and I steps. Review of previous steps will provide insight as to why the behavior or treatment is suggested. Each step of PITS continues to build on the previous step. Repetition of the previous steps covered will reinforce information through conditioning or strengthening associations through the law of exercise (Lefrancois, 1995; Thorndike, 1932) as well as helping to organize the mental connection of new information with present schema (Anderson et al., 1984; Armbruster, 1996; Ormrod, 2008; Shuell, 1990). The repetition of content previously reviewed helps move information along through the three stages of memory noted in section II (Balota and Marsh, 2004).

Until the *S* (specifics) stage, information has been mostly disease or health state centered. Progression to the S stage of PITS moves the instruction toward patient-centered information. Specifics denotes the personalization of treatment. In this stage, the information delivered is tailored specifically for that patient only, hence, patient-specific instruction. During this specific stage, personal medications with individual dosage, diet restrictions only for that patient, and individual activity restrictions are reviewed. This stage cannot be taught to a classroom of patients; this stage is only about one individual, the patient. Like every prior stage, reviewing information from the previous steps, before the addition of specific information for this step, helps to provide material in an orderly and sequential manner. Previous steps should provide a logical foundation for the information that is covered in this stage. Figure 10.4 illustrates the presence of S-R as information transitions from the T stage to the S stage of PITS.

PITS serves as a guide for health material delivery. The patient needs to better understand their disease process to be able to participate in their care and be more than just a recipient of care. The PITS model follows the diagnosing and treatment process (Figure 10.5). For example, a patient presents

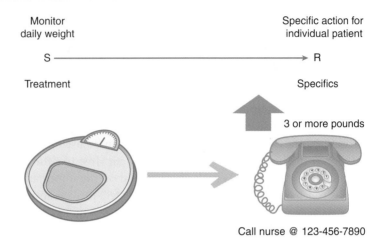

Fig. 10.4   Stimulus-response of treatment to specifics stage of PITS model.
The figure illustrates the relationship of the treatment and specifics to the stimulus-response model. © Melissa N. Stewart.

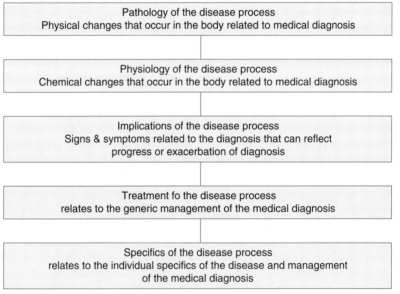

Fig. 10.5   PITS model. The figure offers a quick visual of each step of the PITS model with a brief explanation of the meaning and focus of each step. © Melissa N. Stewart.

with symptoms (indications), the patient is assessed (pathology), lab work is done (physiology), and treatment is ordered (standards of practice) reflecting specifics of individualized needs (personalized individualized care ordered and information needed). PITS serves as a way of communicating with the healthcare consumer throughout the diagnosis, planning, treatment, and maintenance phases of care. The PITS model provides an outline of what, how, and why for the patient, then offers generalized solutions followed by specific solutions. The PITS model serves to define a pathway for information delivery by healthcare providers as they guide healthcare consumers toward their personal healthcare goals.

PITS is not specific to a particular discipline and can be used by any healthcare provider. It is recommended that healthcare providers review each stage in the order of the model even if the intent is to teach information in the last stage.

How Two Different Healthcare Providers Used PITS to Instruct Patient on Self-Care for Congestive Heart Failure

Haddie, the retired cafeteria worker discussed in Chapter 10, needs to learn about her chronic illness: congestive heart failure. The nurse needs to teach her weight parameter triggers for calling the provider, and the phone number to call. The nurse then begins her instruction with a brief review of pathophysiology and indication: "Remember how when the heart is not pumping effectively the body will hold water and may swell" (Indications). "Daily weigh-ins (Treatment) are needed to help identify when the body is holding water before there is a lot of swelling. If you experience a 3-pound or greater weight gain in your morning weight, you will need to call your nurse at this number" (Specifics).

The therapist needs to teach the same patient about safe ambulation. The therapist reviews pathophysiology and indication first: "Remember your heart pump is not effectively working so the body may hold water/swell." He goes on to cover daily weigh-ins (traditional treatment) and their use in identifying when the body is holding water before there is too much swelling. He tells Haddie that she will need to use her walker as she weighs in every morning. He instructs Haddie on how to position the scale so the walker can move over the scale. Once on the scale, the therapist tells Haddie to hold on to the walker until she is balanced. When balanced, he advises her to look at the number then let go, look at number again, then re-grip her walker. He estimates that she should not have to let her walker go for more than a minute. This example demonstrates how healthcare providers from two separate disciplines can teach the same patient using PITS from their practice focus. Figure 10.6 displays the progress of information using PITS in two different disciplines.

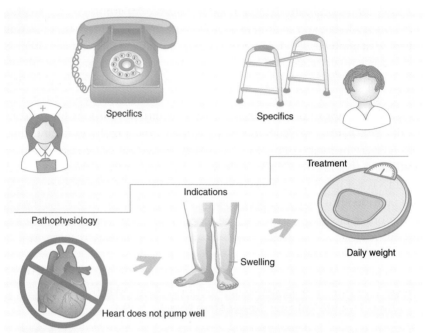

Fig. 10.6 PITS used by different disciplines. The figure displays the combined steps of PITS from the focus of different disciplines. The pathophysiology, indication, and treatment stages of PITS provide the foundation for the specific exercises the physical therapist wants the patient to do while also supporting the phone call the nurse wants the patient to make regarding specific changes in daily weights.

The revisiting of each stage previously covered in PITS serves as a foundation for progression to the next stage, assisting the receiver in the accommodation and assimilation of the new information (Lund et al., 2005; Novak, 1998; Saunders, 1992). Perpetually revisiting information provides reinforcement of the information, which helps to mentally "stamp in" knowledge and progress new data into the long-term memory (Cowan, 2001; MacGregor, 1987; Thorndike, 1932). Each provider delivers information in treatment and specifics framed in the focus of their discipline. For example, nursing may focus on self-care teaching, whereas a dietitian will focus on diet teaching, the doctor may discuss diagnostics needed, the physical therapist will focus on mobility, safety, and exercise, whereas the pharmacist focuses on medication administration. When the information is presented by multiple disciplines in the same manner, it shows the unity of providers toward treatment while offering the benefit of reinforcing information repeatedly. Empowering the patient with information elevates the consumer to a partner with a degree of responsibility in their health.

The first two stages of PITS, PI, should not vary by discipline. The T (treatment) stage is where the variation may begin according to each provider's particular discipline focus on healthcare treatment. For example, a physical therapist who is treating a patient who has received PIT instruction would briefly review pathophysiology and indications, and then focus on specific exercises ordered. The physical therapist may pull from the pathology and indications to correlate the exercises relevant to the symptoms experienced, or to the disease pathology and how the exercises will decrease the problems experienced, or improve physical alterations. This gives meaning and justification to the exercises. It also helps to give direct control to the patient in achievement of optimal health. The patient can directly correlate their activity to improvement in their health condition.

Evaluation of presenting knowledge is easier if the patient's healthcare providers are using PITS. The provider simply needs to evaluate the patient's understanding of each step to see where they are in their understanding. A noticeable deficit in one step should alert the provider to concentrate their efforts on that information step. PITS offers a universal teaching model for all disease processes for all disciplines. From physician to therapist, dietitian to nurse, all disciplines can follow PITS, each adding their discipline's focus on patient treatment. All disciplines can use PITS to relay their information. Each provider focuses on the same disease—each treating and teaching from their discipline, and all building on one another's patient education efforts while improving their patients' knowledge of their health. Providers may never meet, but by using the same model, PITS, they build on each other's educational contributions in their patient population.

Summary

- Information needs to have a logical flow so it can be easily received, filed, and retrieved.
- Information delivered in an orderly fashion makes sense and allows the receiver to easily follow the educator's train of thought.
- Redman (2007) points out that information needs to be delivered in an orderly, sequential style according to the patient's order of need. The author suggests information flow either from disease toward the patient or away from the patient toward disease.

■ The PITS model was created by the author in an attempt to bring order to patient educational efforts. It offers a logical organized format to deliver health or disease state information, resulting in a standard communication methodology for the delivery of patient education. PITS, in a natural state, flows from disease state toward patient; however, it can be inverted to change the flow of information from the patient toward the disease state.

■ PITS is an acronym that serves as a patient education model, a common map or pathway for patient education. The acronym stands for pathophysiology, indications, treatment, and specifics.

■ The P denotes pathophysiology. Pathology includes all that is physical. The pathology is the segment of education in which the educator identifies any physical changes that have or could occur as the result of a disease, condition, insult, or health state.

■ The I in PITS represents indications. Indications are the signs or symptoms that may occur as the result of the disease or health state. Symptoms include what the patient may experience as well as what may be observed or found on assessment. These symptoms may be used as an indicator of disease progression, maintenance, and exacerbation.

■ The PI of PITS serves as the rationale for the reason a treatment is ordered.

■ The T of PITS refers to treatment. Treatment is the gold standard or industry-accepted treatment of the disease or health state for which the provider is treating the patient. In this stage, treatment information specific to the disease or health state is provided. Complex instructions need to be broken down and taught one step at a time.

■ The S refers to specifics. This is the personalization of treatment. In this stage, the information delivered is tailored specifically for that patient only, hence, it is patient-specific instruction. During this specific stage, personal medications with individual dosage, diet restrictions only for that patient, and individual activity restrictions are reviewed.

■ The PITS model provides an outline of what, how, and why for the patient, and then offers generalized solutions followed by specific solutions. The model serves to define a pathway for information delivery by healthcare providers as they guide healthcare consumers toward their personal healthcare goals.

■ PITS is not specific to a particular discipline and can be used by any healthcare provider. It is recommended that healthcare providers review

each stage in the order of the model even if the intent is to teach information in the last stage.

- The revisiting of each stage previously covered in PITS serves as a foundation for progression to the next stage, assisting the receiver in the
accommodation and assimilation of the new information.

- The first two stages of PITS, PI should not vary by discipline. The T
(treatment) stage is where the variation may begin according to the
particular focus of the provider's discipline on healthcare treatment.

- Each provider focuses on the same disease, with each treating and
teaching from their discipline, and all building on one another's patient
education efforts while improving their patients' knowledge of their
health. Providers may never meet, but by using the same model, PITS,
they build on each other's educational contributions in their patient
population.

CHAPTER 11

The Medagogy Conceptual Framework

In healthcare, the provider and the patient should share one guiding common interest: the patient's health. The patient should be the focus of all decisions. All interactions and treatment should be predicated on respect for patients, including their ability and right to know and understand their healthcare treatment, choices, obligations, and commitments. The hope is that healthcare providers are able to meet patients' needs and help patients reach or exceed their personal health goals.

To accomplish this, there must be effective communication between provider and patient as well as between providers. The PITS model discussed in Chapter 10 offers a common pathway for information delivery, exchange, flow, processing, and influence in the decision-making process. The medagogy conceptual framework focuses on the overarching process of patient education while concentrating on the flow and operation of information. This theoretical structure includes the steps of health knowledge gain, the informational seasons of patient education, and the PITS model. This conceptual philosophy is meant to serve as a common framework for information delivery in the daily practice of patient education. Medagogy succinctly communicates the complexities of patient education in healthcare. Figure 11.1 displays the medagogy conceptual framework.

The beauty of this theoretical framework lies in the unlimited possibilities provided by the individual's values and interpretations. However, that great variety also creates a problem when the time comes to implement the conceptual framework. If medagogy is to serve as a common model for a team, then all members of the team need to have a working knowledge of the model and its impact on practice. Just as patients need time to ingest, digest, and reflect on information, the same is true for members of the healthcare team. Once information has been self-interpreted and action ensues, then team members can decide how to put the model into practice as a team.

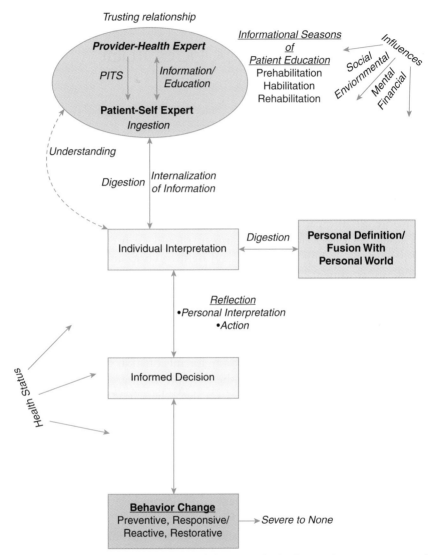

Fig. 11.1 The medagogy conceptual framework. In the medagogy conceptual framework, the flow of information in patient education is displayed as all of the components of patient education are pulled together, from the patient-provider relationship, through internalization of information, to the ultimate behavior changes that result from informed decision making. © Melissa N. Stewart.

Information Movement in Medagogy

The medagogy model provides definition to the process of patient learning by identifying the components of information exchange in the patient education process. Medagogy maintains that patient learning begins with a trusting relationship between healthcare provider and patient. In the provider-patient relationship, the provider serves as the expert of health and the patient serves as the expert of self. A certain level of power comes with expert status.

Healthcare providers have long been comfortable with the power associated with expert status (Shea, 2006). Medagogy asserts that no other person can know more about self than self. Therefore, in the patient-provider relationship, the patient must assume the rightful position as expert of self.

Information flow is continuous between provider and patient. Information exchanged ranges from exposure to instruction and may contain any material from personal facts and data to casual lighthearted dialogue. Treatment directions and suggestions should be formatted so that patients can understand the information, make informed decisions, and follow through with established health plans.

The information exchanged by the patient and the provider is internalized by each. As the internalized information is assimilated, an individual interpretation evolves. With the addition of new information to the patient's personal knowledge base, individual interpretation merges the newly acquired information with the patient's personal world. Once the information is integrated into the patient's personal world, it can be accessed as needed for everyday living. The resulting interpretation helps guide the patient's decision-making process. The same is true for the provider; understanding the unique aspects of a patient enhances the provider's ability to make informed and personalized decisions.

Information reception, processing, and decision-making is affected by the patient's health status and other influences like physical, mental, financial, environmental, and social status along with cultural and spiritual beliefs (Falvo, 1994; Henderson, 2002; Pierce and Hicks, 2001; Prossier et al., 2003; Stewart et al., 2000). Physical phenomena include physical limitations like motor control or ability, vision, hearing, tolerance, and comfort (Stewart et al., 2000). Mental activity influences include learning disabilities, cognitive deficit, and illness or treatment haze where mental clarity is hazy secondary to illness or treatment, as in cases of surgery recovery or pain medication usage (Falvo, 1994; Stewart et al., 2000). Financial influences include financial obligations, limitations, and constraints (Greene and Adelman, 2003; Henderson, 2002). Environmental influences are related to the physical environment of the healthcare setting, personal home, work, and social surroundings (Curtis et al., 2000; Falvo, 1994; Gabbay at al., 2000). Social influences include social networks, community, culture, and the attitudes of family and friends, in addition to accepted and adopted norms (Kravitz et al., 2002). Spiritual influences include personal, cultural, and faith-based beliefs and values (Falvo, 1994; Greene and Adelman, 2003).

Certified patient educators (CPEs) offer invaluable expertise to the healthcare team that is committed to addressing patient literacy in their practice. CPEs trained in the medagogy model played an integral role in the success of the Centers for Medicare and Medicaid Services (CMS) care transitions pilot. In the care transitions pilot, CPEs initiated as per medagogy model a structured patient education plan for each patient that was accepted into project. They managed a population of patients' knowledge needs as the patients safely transitioned from acute (dependent care) to home (self/independent care), along with assisting patients to successfully meet their treatment plan goals, inclusive of follow-up healthcare access. Together, the CPEs and their extender, the Patient Specialist (PS-c), helped their patients avoid readmission and inappropriate resource utilization.

A CPE can be requested to evaluate a patient, or a protocol can require all admitted patients to be evaluated by a CPE. Evaluation needs to include the patient's learning style (primary and secondary), ideal time of day for learning, admitting level of knowledge, learning disabilities, need for learning aides, and the patient's perception of his learning needs. Working within a trusting relationship, identified in the conceptual model for medagogy, the patient educator, as an expert of health, exchanges information with the patient, who is recognized as the expert of self. The informational seasons discussed previously help the CPE deliver information according to the patient's health positioning. Figure 11.2 represents positioning of health in life. After assessment and information exchange, the CPE can draft a teaching plan that includes learning objectives, teaching materials to be used, methods of instruction, and modes of evaluating comprehension, which aligns team members' contributions.

After the teaching plan is drafted, it can then serve as a form of communication between providers regarding the patient's progress toward health knowledge. The teaching plan transitions into a report card system that can flow between providers as each one contributes to the plan. The report card system serves as a tool to communicate progress, but also contains an assessment of the patient's learning needs. With a quick glance, each provider can determine how best to deliver information to the patient. The report card also provides insight into the patient's strengths and weaknesses regarding knowledge. The report card should be a never-ending, living document that follows the patient throughout the healthcare system. As patients transition

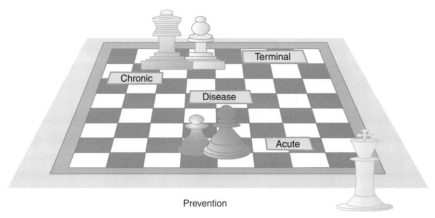

Fig. 11.2   Patients' personal positioning regarding health. The illustration displays the personal positioning of individuals with regard to their health throughout life.

between providers and care settings, they are exposed to copious health-sustaining information that is often lost, misunderstood, or undervalued. Just as physical care alterations are exchanged between healthcare settings and healthcare providers, patient health knowledge should also progress through the system with the patient. New objectives and teaching methods are added as the patient's knowledge and/or health status changes. Figure 11.3 displays the report card exchange as it moves through various providers.

The CPE or designated patient educator can periodically evaluate the patient's comprehension to provide a common, consistent provider evaluation. In addition, learning boosters or refreshers from occasional educational sessions can help a patient who is not actively engaged in healthcare delivery continue to avoid the need to access healthcare because of acute episodic symptomology. By refreshing the patient's memory with previously reviewed information, previously stored information can be reactivated and information that may not have made it into long-term memory can work through the stages of memory. Reexposure to information helps to reenergize stored information (Zull, 2006). It is easier to relearn information forgotten or not retained (Sousa, 2006). This memory refresher provides a mental boost of information for the patient so that information does not become stagnant or stale, which may lead to nonuse of needed information and/or decreased exactness of the information (Feldman and McPhee, 2008; Ormrod, 2008). Engaging patients when they are not in a crisis or an acute health situation helps to reenergize the neural forests discussed in Chapter 9 and awaken patients' consciousness of their health while, hopefully, providing a less emotionally challenging teaching opportunity (Zull, 2006).

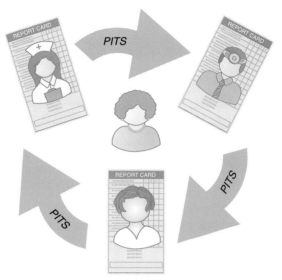

Fig. 11.3   Illustration of provider report card system. Information exchange between providers is accomplished by using a report card system. The patient and the certified patient educator serve as a hub for the patient's present level of understanding and progression of knowledge.

Ingestion to Digestion

Once information is received or ingested, the breakdown of the information, or mental digestion, begins. Digestion in the gastrointestinal system of the body involves the chemical and physical breakdown of ingested food. The food is separated, then stored or discarded according to how the body will need or use it. The mental ingestion and digestion of information is very similar to the gastrointestinal process. Information received is internalized, or taken in, through ingestion. In the digestion of information, personal values and beliefs help in the personal interpretation of information. Who, how, when, and where all play a part in influencing personal perception of information.

Personal definition involves individual values and beliefs along with the personal world, which includes social support systems and social interactions like family, friends, and job. In the book *Through the Patient's Eyes*, attention is drawn to the need for healthcare providers to be respectful of patients' life experiences, culture, and beliefs, including the impacts of these on healthcare decision-making (Gerteis et al., 1993). Medagogy attempts to capture the effect of individualism in the medagogic process of interpretation resulting from fusion of new information with the personal world. The personal world is a conglomeration of all the intricacies of personal life including recreational activities like exercise and hobbies, as well as faith-based convictions and political practices. Fishbein and Ajzen (1975) acknowledge in their predictive persuasion theory, discussed in Chapter 5, that personal beliefs influence a person's behavior. Pender et al. (2002) capture the concept of medagogy in the personal world in their health promotion model as interpersonal influences. If something is important enough for the patient to participate in regularly, it is of value to the patient. Even if participation is a requirement of a relationship, the follow-through of participation is representative of worth. The worth of participation may be based in the value of the relationship.

How Laurie's Values Affect Her Decision?

Laurie, a professor at the local college, and her husband Jim, a local plumber, faithfully attend all of the football games at the local college. Laurie does not like football, but the event is not the impetus of her action. The relationship with her spouse is where the value lies. So why would this be important in health? Health can impact how people live life. The better patients feel, the more they are able to live life without unhealthy inhibition. Health can divert personal life temporarily or permanently. For example, the acute and temporary health change of a broken leg may make attendance at football games impossible for the remainder of the season, whereas a diagnosis of muscular dystrophy may gradually decrease the physical stamina required for football game attendance as a permanent and chronic health alteration. Health behavior choices are influenced by individual interpretation, which is perpetually affected by one's personal world.

Individuals do not determine the value of all information internally. Some information is deemed of personal worth in concert with external influences at the time of ingestion, digestion, and reflection. Health status is a major external influence on the patient's mental processing of information. Health status reflects where patients are on their health continuum. A fever with head congestion may influence the ingestion of information. The congestion may decrease the ability to hear what is being said, whereas the fever may cause a distracted mentality that could influence the processing of information. Medications and health indications can decrease alertness, affecting the patient's ability to mentally file information and successfully move through the stages of memory (short to long term). Health status also refers to Bishop's (1991) suggestion that patients make their own mental representation of any alteration in health. Simpson et al. (1991) discuss the variance in perceptions between provider and patient, including illness perceptions.

Part of the disparity is related to varying illness representations, which can be attributed to individualism as well as to internal and external influences like health (Skevington and Garro, 1995; Weinman et al., 1996).

Environmental influences relate to the physical environment of the healthcare setting and the person's home, work, and social surroundings. When educating the patient, the environment where the patient is taught can influence learning (Falvo, 1994; Redman, 2007). A patient educator can evaluate physical surroundings using his senses: visual, auditory, tactile, taste, and even smell. The setting in which the healthcare information is delivered might be noisy, with competing sounds that interfere with receiving information. The setting may contain visual distractions, making it difficult for the patient to focus on the message. Senses like touch, taste, and smell bear mentioning because they have influencing power. The sense of touch determines if the environment is comfortable; consider the room's physical temperature or seating, as well as the general physical comfort of the patient. The sense of smell can physically impact a person. For example, noxious smells can be distracting, whereas some aromas can be stimulating and make a person more receptive to learning. Some treatments can cause a bad taste in the mouth, which can be a negative distraction. Environment may also include conditions like the provider-patient relationship. The provider-patient relationship can be influenced by a patient's desire to please the provider; it can also cause dissatisfaction and distrust in a patient (Heisler et al., 2002). The environmental influence of the provider's healthcare decision-making style will determine if the provider is open to patient inclusion in the treatment planning process (Guadagnoli and Ward, 1998; Van de Borne, 1998). A cooperative partnership environment will encourage and support patient involvement in making healthcare decisions (Guadagnoli and Ward, 1998).

Fishbein and Ajzen's (1975) predictive persuasion theory accounts for the social environment's influence on a person's behavior. Medagogy also acknowledges the impact that social influence may have on patient health decisions and, ultimately, patient actions. Social influence is so important that it is captured both in internal and external influences. Beyond the internal composition of one's personal world as an external influence, social influences include cultural and social networks, community, the attitudes of family and friends, as well as accepted and adopted norms.

Medagogy attempts to determine social influences of which the patient may not even be aware. External social influences may occur through subconscious conditioning (as discussed under Behaviorism in Chapter 4) via social norms that have meshed with the self over time.

How Childhood Caused a Lingering Health Bias in Adulthood

External social influence is noted in the following example of assumed passivity in the patient role. Like many people, Bob, an ex-Marine, was told to take his medicine when he was a child. He was also told to be quiet when the doctors, as well as other adults, were talking. Young Bob went to the doctor for boosters, vaccinations, and when he was not feeling well. Over time, Bob was conditioned to dread doctor visits and to passively follow his doctors' advice without question. Not all people assume the level of passivity that Bob acquired over time. Bob internalized and accepted certain social influences as a child; Bob's passivity in the patient role is a lingering bias he still carries in his adulthood. Bob's decisions in his healthcare will be made in the presence of this personal bias.

External mental influence is captured as presenting knowledge and the ability to acquire knowledge. Presenting knowledge may be in any subject matter, including but not limited to health. As discussed in Bloom's taxonomy in Chapter 5, the question for the healthcare provider is whether the patient is able to create or whether they remember. The ability to acquire knowledge involves the patient's learning style and preferences, including capabilities and limitations, as well as the patient's circadian rhythm for learning. For example, is the patient a morning learner or an evening learner? Learning capabilities and limitations include learning disabilities, history of learning successes and failures, cognitive deficit, and illness or treatment haze affecting mental clarity (such as surgery recovery or pain medication usage). Refer to Chapter 5 for a detailed discussion of learning styles.

Financial influences like financial obligations, limitations, and constraints are also external influences. Financial influences can be profoundly distracting for a patient. A patient's concern about treatment cost can induce feelings of fear and anxiety, which can impact patient decision-making. Financial impact can also limit treatment choices because of a patient's personal financial constraints. Piette et al. (2004) surveyed 660 Americans about medication cost. Survey findings revealed that 440 of those surveyed confessed that they underuse their prescribed medications because of cost and they have never told their healthcare provider. Interestingly, 435 of the survey respondents also reported that they have never been asked if they can afford their prescribed medication (Piette et al., 2004). Another financial concern well documented in the literature is the healthcare provider's personal financial gain related to the prescribed treatment, pointing to the question of patient versus personal interests affecting treatment decisions (Emaneul and Goldman, 1998; Levinson et al., 1999).

How Financial Limitations Affect Decision About a Kidney Transplant

John, a 64-year-old male patient, is a local businessman who needs a kidney transplant. John does not have health insurance and cannot afford to pay for the organ transplant. John's financial status limits his treatment options and excludes the transplant option from his menu of treatment choices.

Reflection of knowledge begins to become apparent in the transition from personal interpretation to informed decision. All of the previous factors and their influencing powers are present in the informed decision. The degree to which they are acknowledged or used is personal, but their presence is there. The presence of these other factors offers insight into why the patient should have an understanding of the information influencing the healthcare provider's treatment decisions. Without their providers' information concerning pathophysiology, indications, textbook treatment, and individual specifics, patients can rely only on what they already know. Not knowing the pathophysiology, indications, textbook treatment, and individual specifics limits the patient's ability to make an informed decision. Knowing these things balances the decision with health knowledge.

Lack of Mechanical Knowledge Causes Car Engine to Die

Lulu, a local housewife, has no knowledge about how cars work. She brings her car to a shop because it has been making a strange noise. The mechanic queries her, then looks at the engine and the underside of the car. The mechanic tells Lulu that she will need a $2000 engine repair. Lulu asks "Why?" The mechanic replies, "Because the car engine is sick." Lulu then asks for an explanation. The mechanic explains the problem with the car using mechanical terminology like piston, head gasket, crankshaft, and cylinder head. The mechanic hears a bell, signaling the next client's arrival and hurriedly tells Lulu, "You just think about it and let me know what you decide." Before he can leave her, Lulu asks, "What will happen if I do not get the work done that you recommend?" The mechanic responds, "The car will die," as he hands her a bill, tells her to pay the lady at the window on her way out, and then walks away. Dazed and confused, Lulu immediately tries to call her best friend to get advice as she makes her way to the payment window. Lulu's best friend tells her not to worry, that her sister's car did the same thing and it just went away. She advises Lulu to forget about it and not to let the mechanic take advantage of her. Lulu takes her best friend's advice and the car stalls just two blocks from the mechanic's shop. Mechanical knowledge of the problem could have helped Lulu balance her decision-making with knowledge she is unaware of, the information the mechanic was using to make his mechanical diagnosis.

Decisions that patients make reflect their interpretation of the situation, values, influencing factors, and understanding. If the decision is made with accurate understanding of the pathophysiology of the health status, indications, treatment, and specifics, then the patient has made an informed decision. Action occurs based on the patient's decision. Medagogy focuses on the action of behavior change. Behavior change may be severe, such as a complete change from presenting behavior and lifestyle. For example, consider a cardiac, overweight, and sedentary person who decides to diet and exercise daily to improve his heart health. No change would mean the cardiac patient decides not to make any lifestyle changes, including medication administration. No change in behavior is still considered an action because it represents choice. Whatever the patient's decision, as long as the provider has made health information available and understandable to the patient, then the healthcare provider should respect the patient's choice. The healthcare provider should always make the information that they are using to guide health treatment decisions available to the patient even if the patient has chosen not to change behavior.

Behavior change that does occur in response to informed decision may be preventive, responsive or reactive, or restorative. These behavior changes are reflective of the patient's informational season (see Chapter 8). The prehabilitative informational season of patient education involves the delivery of information to a patient at risk for an insult to health. The behavior change that is associated with this informational season is prevention. Preventive behavior change occurs before an insult to health. The focus of prevention is to avoid negative health status. The goal is for prehabilitative education to yield preventive behavior change in the patient. Once an insult to health has occurred, the patient then enters the habilitation informational season. In habilitation, the information is focused on developing new lifestyle habits to help control health status and to avoid negative health outcomes. Responsive or reactive behavior change occurs in response to a negative change in health status. The behavior change is warranted to control, or to try to control, the health state. The rehabilitation informational season focuses educational efforts on helping the patient regain any loss that has occurred as the result of negative health status. Restorative behavior change occurs in response to a negative health occurrence. Behavior is focused on restoring health to a pre-insult health state. Figure 11.4 displays the relationship of the informational seasons to patient behavior change.

Medagogy serves as a model to connect all of the elements of the patient education process, from information delivery to action. Medagogy views informational processing in patient education from the patient's perspective.

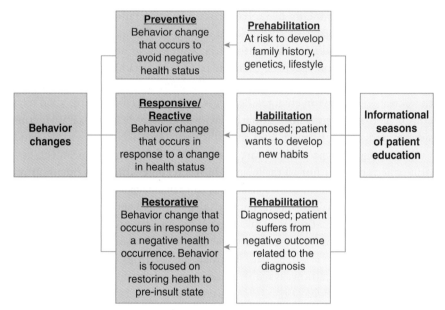

Fig. 11.4 The informational seasons of patient education. The informational seasons of patient education are related to the types of behavior changes they can produce. © Melissa N. Stewart.

Medagogy's conceptual framework begins with the initial exchange between two experts: provider, the expert of health, and patient, the expert of self, through the internalization of information. Informational seasons of patient education help orient information to a patient's present health status in relation to health concerns identified by the healthcare provider. Information delivered to the patient initiates movement toward acquiring health knowledge. Along the path of gaining knowledge, internal and external personal influences are encountered as the patient begins to merge the health state with self. The individualism of understanding is revealed in reflection, where action occurs based on the patient's informed decision. The medagogy model attempts to communicate the many facets involved in patients' processing of provided information and the impacts of their perceptions on decision making.

Constructing Information for Delivery to Patients

Once a patient's learning styles and preferences are identified, they should become part of the patient's health demographic information. As a provider plans to educate a patient, he should reference the patient's education hierarchy as well as the informational seasons of patient education. After the patient's informational season and level on the hierarchy are identified, the patient educator needs to choose a method of delivery for patient information. Before information delivery, the method for evaluating patient understanding should be identified. Once these key pieces are in place, education can begin. The purpose of the teaching intervention should be clear to both patient and provider before initiation so that a level of achievement can be determined.

Medagogy offers a glimpse into the patient's learning process versus traditional healthcare initiatives that are more provider-centered, focusing on what will be delivered and when it will be delivered. Instead of working the patient into healthcare provider plans, medagogy invites providers to step back and move with the patient rather than being two steps ahead of them. This is not to say the medagogy model must be used independently.

As evidenced in the community-based care transitions program (CCTP) of the Affordable Healthcare Act, medagogy can beautifully complement successful projects like RED (Reengineering Hospital Discharge) and BOOST (Better Outcomes for Older Adults through Safe Transitions). Either project can be implemented with medagogy concepts to help providers deliver patient-centered communication while harnessing the full power of individual patient education efforts. Interdependently and/or independently, medagogy can assist providers as they help their patients gain physical and mental control of their health.

Summary

- In healthcare, the provider and the patient should both share one guiding common interest: the patient's health. The patient should be the focus of all decisions.

- To accomplish this, there must be effective communication between provider and patient as well as between providers. The PITS model (see Chapter 10) offers a common pathway for information delivery, exchange, flow, processing, and influence in the decision-making process.

- If medagogy is to serve as a common model for a team, then all members of the team need to have a working knowledge of the model and its impact on practice.

- Certified patient educators (CPEs) offer invaluable expertise to the healthcare team that is committed to addressing patient literacy in their practice.

- After assessment and information exchange, the patient educator can begin to draft a teaching plan including learning objectives, teaching materials to be used, methods of instruction, modes of evaluation of comprehension, and names of responsible providers.

- After the teaching plan is drafted, it can serve as a form of communication between providers regarding the patient's progress toward health knowledge.

- A CPE or designated patient educator can periodically perform evaluations of comprehension to provide a common, consistent provider evaluation.

- Once information is received or ingested, the breakdown of the information or mental digestion begins. The mental ingestion and digestion of information is very similar to the gastrointestinal process. Information received is internalized, or taken in, through ingestion.

- When educating the patient, the environment where the patient is taught can influence learning. A patient educator can evaluate physical surroundings using his own senses: visual, auditory, tactile, taste, and even smell.

- Environment may include the condition of the provider-patient relationship. The provider-patient relationship can be influenced by a patient's desire to please the provider; it can also cause dissatisfaction and distrust in a patient.

- Financial influences like financial obligations, limitations, and constraints are considered external influences. Financial influences can be profoundly distracting for a patient.

- Not knowing the pathophysiology, indications, textbook treatment, and individual specifics limits the patient's ability to make an informed decision. Knowing these things balances the decision with health knowledge.

- The decisions that patients make are a reflection of their interpretation of the situation, values, influencing factors, and understanding.

- Whatever a patient's decision, as long as the provider has made health information available and understandable to the patient, then the healthcare provider should respect the patient's choice.

- Behavior change that occurs in response to informed decision-making may be preventive, responsive or reactive, or restorative.

- The medagogy model serves to connect all of the elements in the patient education process, from information delivery to action. Medagogy views informational processing in patient education from the patient's perspective.

- The conceptual framework of medagogy begins with the initial exchange between two experts: provider, the expert of health, and patient, the expert of self, through the internalization of information.
- Once patients' learning styles and preferences are identified, they should become part of their health demographic information.
- The purpose of the teaching intervention should be clear to both patient and provider before initiation so a level of achievement can be determined.
- Medagogy can complement successful projects such as RED (Reengineering Hospital Discharge) and BOOST (Better Outcomes for Older Adults through Safe Transitions).

CHAPTER 12

Assessing Patient Knowledge Using The Understanding Personal Perception Tool

As healthcare becomes more patient oriented, providers must treat each patient as an individual. The aspiration of a new patient-oriented community of care can only become reality by addressing each patient's health literacy needs. Through a structured approach to patient education and communication, providers can unite their efforts and progressively add to each individual patient's health knowledge reservoir.

The report of the Institute of Medicine (IOM, 2004) has suggested that all health professions engage in program activities that emphasize respect for, and understanding of, cultural and individual patient and family diversity (Smedley et al., 2004). The IOM further emphasizes that personal and demographic characteristics such as age, disability, ethnicity, gender, language, national origin, religion, sexual orientation, and socioeconomic status be considered when planning all aspects of patient care. Importantly, this approach must also include patient education. The medagogy model emphasizes cultural and individual diversity and reinforces the assumption that every human being is uniquely different (M. Jewell, personal communication, March 10, 2010).

The medagogy framework offers a pathway for educating individuals that can be beneficial in chronic illness management and care coordination. Treatment and management of chronic illness translates financially into more than $1 trillion dollars of the annual US federal healthcare budget (Wagner, 2004). It is imperative that self-care and self-management be buttressed in all patient education teachings, especially for those individuals with chronic health conditions. According to Wagner (2004), 95% of the Medicare budget is spent on chronic illness. Two-thirds of the 65 years of age and older population lives with four or more chronic health conditions; prevention along with improved self-care and self-management can help preserve the limited healthcare resources of our nation, both human and fiscal (Wagner, 2004). A healthier nation of people as a result of informed engagement in self-care is a realistic and noble goal.

Knowledge Measurement

Patient education should include evaluative techniques to assess patient understanding (Redman, 2003). Historically, standard knowledge measurement that is traditional to academic settings has not been used in healthcare. Tests and quizzes and performance-based assessments of knowledge are not a common practice in patient education (Falvo, 1994; Lainscak and Keber, 2005; Redman, 2001, 2003). Instead, in patient education a loose qualitative labeling suffices as the "norm" for knowledge evaluation (Escalante et al., 2004; Freeman and Chambers, 1997). For instance, if a patient is exposed to health information, the healthcare provider may document "able to verbalize understanding" or "able to repeat back" (Escalante et al., 2004; Freeman and Chambers, 1997). Neither of these examples, however, offers insight as to where the patient is in their knowledge attainment. The first example, "able to verbalize understanding" could possibly even be a brush-off from the patient like, "of course, I got it." The second example, "able to repeat back," is commonly seen in exotic birds and parrots, which is why parroting is a fitting label for this sort of appraisal. Neither example hits the mark of identifying the patient's status in learning, nor does either example give the healthcare provider the ability to understand a patient's grasp of information.

Providers need a systematic approach to use in evaluating and following a patient's knowledge gain as they strive to move patients toward greater health awareness and independence. Vague and limited provider insight, at best, is achieved through present patient education evaluation methods. Capturing the progression of patient knowledge and intervening when knowledge deficits put the patient at risk can help the patient avoid unnecessary health setbacks as well as inappropriate or avoidable resource utilization. Perpetually increasing the patient's knowledge as he moves throughout the healthcare system will advance the patient toward independent self-care, health sustainability, and health autonomy.

Need for a Patient Perception Tool

Universally, health literacy definitions acknowledge patients' needs to understand and use health information to which they have been exposed. Feldman and McPhee (2008) acknowledge that comprehension and understanding are abstract; therefore, direct measurement is often challenging. Although instruments serve as a form of assessment to determine the level of understanding of a subject or content, results can be misleading. Fears, poor test-taking skills, low reading literacy, the quality of items on the measurement tools or instruments, and sometimes poorly selected variables can affect test results. The results could misrepresent a person's understanding of information which translates, in clinical practice, to insufficient self-care information.

To determine the state of the science, Stewart conducted a literature review which revealed that a number of measures have been developed to assess patient knowledge. The Michigan Diabetes Research Training Centers (MDRTC) diabetes knowledge test consists of 23 multiple-choice questions (Fitzgerald et al., 1998; Redman, 2003). Approximately 15 minutes is required to complete the MDTRC knowledge test (Redman, 2003). Reliability and validity were first collected in a study of 811 participants from two different Michigan communities; one community received at-home services for their diabetes care (312 subjects), while the second community received diabetes care in a Michigan Department of Public Health clinical setting (499 subjects). The two sample populations were similar in diabetes type, treatment, years since diagnosis, and academic education completed. The populations varied in age, gender, ethnicity, and previous diabetic education. The public health clinic population included fewer Caucasians, more females, younger participants, and fewer subjects having received previous diabetic education. Although population demographics varied, the populations were found to be similar in sample characteristics. The MDRTC diabetes knowledge test was found to be reliable with a Cronbach's alpha of ≥0.70 on test items (Fitzgerald et al., 1998). At the same time, the MDRTC diabetes knowledge tool is unable to identify specific components of knowledge and self-care due to its generality (Redman, 2003).

The Arthritis Community Research and Evaluation Unit (ACREU) Rheumatoid Arthritis Knowledge Inventory involves 31 statements that are ranked from strongly agree (1) to strongly disagree (5) (Lineker et al., 1997; Redman, 2003). The ACREU knowledge tool inventories knowledge in seven areas identified as learning issues by members of a focus group of individuals with rheumatoid arthritis (Lineker et al., 1997). After the tool was constructed, it was tested for reliability and validity in a population of 252 patients with rheumatoid arthritis in community-based rehabilitation programs or ambulatory or clinical healthcare settings (Lineker et al., 1997; Redman, 2003). More knowledge is indicated through higher scores, and the highest possible score is 31 (Redman, 2003). In populations of people with rheumatoid arthritis, the instrument was found to have acceptable internal consistency with a Cronbach's alpha of 0.76 and a test-retest reliability of 0.92 over 6.7 days (Lineker et al., 1997). A review of the literature revealed that three studies have been conducted using the ACREU tool (Lineker et al., 1997; Lineker, 2001; Bell et al., 1998).

The asthma general knowledge questionnaire for adults (AGKQA) is used to evaluate an adult's knowledge of asthma concepts taught in an educational program. The tool was developed by Allen, Jones, and Oldenburg (Allen and Jones, 1998). According to the SMOG readability formula, AGKQA is written at a 5 grade to 6 grade level (Allen and Jones, 1998). The instrument consists of 31 true or false questions; answers may be true, false, or not sure. Not sure answers are used to prevent guessing the correct answer. Only correct true or false answers are given points; not sure and wrong answers are not allotted any points. The total number of correct answers serves as the total score; hence, scores range from 0 to 31. Questions are separated into five content areas, but no subscales are contained in the instrument. The AGKQA was administered to five volunteers to obtain an estimate for time needed to complete the instrument. Completion of the tool takes approximately 5 to 8 minutes. The AGKQA has an internal consistency of 0.56 at baseline (preinstruction) and 0.80 immediately postinstruction (Redman, 2003). A review of the literature revealed the AGKQA has been used in two studies.

The cardiac knowledge questionnaire (CKQ) has 30 true or false questions in the main body (basic cardiac knowledge scale [BCKS]) with an additional 15 lifestyle questions (cardiac lifestyle knowledge scale [CLKS]) and 10 misconception questions (cardiac misconceptions scale [CMS]) for a total of 55 items in the measure (Lidell and Fridlund, 1996; Maeland and Havik, 1987). The BCKS and the CLKS together form the total cardiac knowledge scale (TCKS) whereas the CMS is separate (Redman, 2003). Content validity for the TCKS was obtained by patients and healthcare professionals, but the 10 CMS questions have not received any measure of validity (Redman, 2003). In a 1987 study, the internal consistency of the CKQ tool was determined as BCKS = 0.84, CLKS = 0.69, and CMS = 0.74 (Redman, 2003). A population of 383 postmyocardial infarct patients were used in the original CKQ tool study (Maeland and Havik, 1987). Subjects who did poorly on the misconception questions were found to have decreased expectations of regaining preinsult independence and had an increased likelihood of readmission for chest pain not related to cardiac insult (Maeland and Havik, 1987, 1988, 1989). For a period of time, patient education appeared to decrease misconceptions; without educational reinforcement, the false impressions returned (Maeland and Havik, 1987, 1988). A literature review found that nine studies have used the CKQ tool to obtain further empirical data.

Increased Interest in Evaluation

Redman (2003) acknowledges that since the publication of the first edition of her book, *Measurement Tools in Patient Education*, which contained 52 instruments, the number of instruments in patient education has almost doubled. She credits this proliferation of new measurement tools to the movement of healthcare toward evidence-based practice. One outgrowth of this movement is enhanced interest in patient education or health literacy.

The use of formal assessments and evaluation tools for patient understanding about various phenomena is not standard practice in healthcare (Falvo, 2004; Redman, 2003). Reluctance to use evaluative tools may be attributed to the time commitment of the provider who would be responsible for teaching, administering, and interpreting the results of the intervention (Redman, 2003). In addition, little information about the teacher and the learner, learning conditions, number of teaching or training interactions, testing, and the amount of time involved in teaching is included in the publications of the instrument and measurement tool studies. This observation is a common finding across the literature that addresses health literacy in acute and community-based settings. In the future, for health literacy to be effective among a diverse patient population, sensitive attention must be given to the development of measures and instruments that are clinically relevant, culturally competent, scientifically robust, and easy to administer, score, and interpret.

Perception in Evaluation

Beyond content intake lies the receiver's comfort with the information and his self-perceived level of mastery. In healthcare, a glimpse into the patient's perception of his understanding of information offers the provider an opportunity to determine where the patient thinks his own knowledge exists on some continuum. Insight into personal perceptions can help the healthcare provider determine what the patient has mastered as well as the areas of deficit. Based on this data, the healthcare provider can develop an intervention that is specific, targeted, and culturally relevant for the patient. Insight into a patient's perception of his ability can help the provider establish a safe environment through appropriate and timely resource utilization. In addition, a provider can note the patient's overall understanding of, and comfort level with, the disease and the prescribed health-promotion activities.

The Wong-Baker pain scale is a visual tool that provides a medium for patients to communicate their perceived level of pain to healthcare providers and other interested parties. The scale was developed to move beyond the healthcare provider's utilization of observation and personal opinion as an assessment of patients' pain levels. It was specifically thought to be helpful when providing services to pediatric patients, who often have a limited ability to articulate details about their pain and its myriad manifestations. The scale uses six faces that range from a smiling happy face at level 0 to a crying face at level 6 (Wong and Baker, 1988). In practice, the Wong-Baker pain scale is a commonly used tool that serves as a standard method for pain assessment across many population groups. The Wong-Baker tool offers a proven, reliable patient perception tool to communicate patients' pain intensity (Kim and Buschmann, 2006; Jansen, 2008; Stubby, 1998). Qualities of the Wong-Baker pain scale such as convenience and portability are inviting for clinicians in practice.

The same simple utility of the Wong-Baker pain scale, if translated into a tool for patient communication of personal perception in understanding and ability, could revolutionize patient education efforts. An understanding of patients' perceptions of their own knowledge and the extent to which they feel able to act could help to improve resource utilization, which has national and global implications. When patient and provider accurately communicate and respect each other, results could include more informed decisions by the patient and the provider, a lower cost of care, and improved mortality and morbidity rates in local and global populations. To this end, the understanding personal perception (UPP) scale has been developed.

Understanding Personal Perception Scale

The UPP scale was created to offer an alternative method of communicating with patients regarding their level or depth of understanding about particular phenomena related to their health status. It shares the visual feature of a Likert scale measurement that is evident in the Wong-Baker scale (Wong and Baker, 1988). The tool was designed using the sun to represent clarity and clearness, and clouds to represent fuzziness of information and/or confusion about the topic being discussed. Figure 12.1 displays the UPP scale. The sun portrays indepth understanding of information related to the health condition, whereas the clouds represent questions and lack of clarity. The sun and cloud images are fashioned in a stair-step manner that is symbolic of upward progression, indicating personal understanding and a sense of self-efficacy. Each step is a numbered point on the five-point Likert scale.

The top level of the scale, level 1, has an image of the sun with no clouds; the correlation is that patients have a comfortable understanding of, or significant clarity about, the content that was introduced in the teaching intervention.

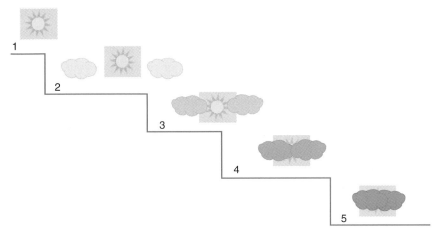

Fig. 12.1 **The understanding personal perception scale.** The sun is representative of clarity of information. The clouds represent confusion, questions, and doubt about the information. © Melissa N. Stewart.

In the downward movements, the steps on the scale have cloud images that are intended to indicate a lack of clarify or the incapacity to "understand or see clearly." Notice that the clouds darken and move toward each other, concealing the sun and limiting clarity or the capacity to "see clearly" as the numbers on the scale move downward toward level 5. Ambiguity, the lack of self-efficacy, and limited understanding of the phenomena would be the interpretation of the patient's level of health literacy if level 5 is indicated. On the other hand, the sun, with its entire array of light, suggests that patients' health literacy is high, that self-efficacy is evident, and that self-care could be safely implemented.

As seen in Figure 12.1, clouds are used to represent some level of confusion, lack of understanding, questions, or lack of clarity. The darker the clouds are, the greater the confusion and lack of clarity. Another factor associated with the clouds is the need for resources. The closer and darker the clouds are and the less the sun is seen, the greater the need for assistance through resources. At level 1, complete sun and no clouds require no resources; the patient is completely independent with the information. Resource requirement increases with movement down toward level 5. At the bottom of the scale, complete dependence on healthcare resources is required. Knowing where patients see themselves in their understanding and ability to act provides insight for the healthcare provider that can be used to safely transition the patient toward an independent state of self-care.

The UPP tool strives to measure the two common themes consistently identified in health literacy: the patient's understanding and the patient's ability to act. The tool uses two questions that the provider asks, and the patient is then instructed to point to their answer on the UPP scale. The first question posed to the patient is, "How clear is your present understanding of this information, previously reviewed with or provided to you?" The patient's answer lets providers know if they can build on present understanding or if they need to clear up any misunderstanding by focusing on areas where there is lack of clarity. The second question is, "How comfortable are you with your understanding and ability to act on or carry out this information?" It is expected that a lack of understanding may influence patients' perceptions of their ability to act. Surprisingly, action is not always contingent on understanding, but action without understanding can pose safety risks. Lack of understanding can serve as a barrier to successful problem solving if any of the patient's circumstances change.

Using the UPP Tool to Help Patient, Monitor Weight

Consider Haddie, the retired cafeteria worker who was being trained by her healthcare providers in Chapter 9. As the healthcare providers train Haddie, they use the UPP tool to capture Haddie's perception of her understanding as well as her comfort with carrying out the new behavior. The nurse walks Haddie through the instruction, has her weigh in, and then reviews the parameters of weight gain that should trigger the need for Haddie to call her provider. At that point, the nurse stops to ask Haddie to use the UPP tool to identify where she feels she is in her understanding. While holding up the tool, the nurse asks Haddie, "How clear is your present understanding of this information I reviewed with you?" Haddie reveals that she's at a level 3 in understanding how to weigh herself and a level 4 regarding when to call. The nurse then asks, "How comfortable are you with your understanding and ability to do this by yourself?" Haddie gives herself a 4 in weighing and a 5 in calling.

By using the UPP tool, the healthcare provider gained insight into Haddie's perception of her understanding and ability to act upon the new information. This information can help the healthcare provider become aware of the resources the patient needs to assist her in carrying out the activity.

The nurse, in collaboration with the patient, decides to follow up with Haddie in a call to review information and walk Haddie through each step of the weigh and call process. The next day, the nurse calls at the established time. Haddie is able to successfully weigh herself and correctly determines that she is not in the parameters that would trigger a phone call to report weight gain. The nurse then asks Haddie to rescale herself using the UPP tool. Haddie picks up the copy of the UPP tool the nurse gave her. On reevaluation, Haddie scales her understanding at 2 and her ability to act at 2. The nurse makes sure Haddie has her contact number and tells Haddie that she will call her next week to ask how things are going. The following week's call reveals that Haddie has been successful in her weight monitoring.

Beyond the Bedside

One of the challenges associated with health literacy is how best to communicate with patients and connect with their personal view within the context of improving health. The UPP scale provides unique insight into where patients envision their understanding and ability to act upon their understanding. Although the conception of the UPP scale originated in healthcare as a tool to be used between the patient and the provider, its use is not limited to the healthcare setting. Portability and ease of use make the tool attractive in other settings. The UPP tool can be used with any information, in any setting, and for any person. The design of the UPP tool allows it to be administered in minimal time, ideally in less than a minute. From the academic classroom to the hospital room, anywhere clear communication and understanding is needed, the tool can be used. Within the healthcare setting, patient satisfaction, effectiveness of patient teaching, and many unseen factors may become apparent with insight into patient perception.

There is abundant evidence to support the benefits that patient education brings to health outcomes (Falvo, 2004; Osborne, 2005; Redman, 2004). Redman (2003) mentions that patient education is routinely practiced in the healthcare setting without a common methodology or approach, and that healthcare system changes will necessitate system-wide recognition of a universal methodical approach to patient education. In the Centers for Medicare and Medicaid Services (CMS) care transitions pilot program, the UPP scale helped certified patient educators and patient specialist coaches identify appropriate follow-up time frames. Recognizing where patients saw themselves in knowledge and ability aided in transitioning patients into self-care safely. The UPP scale provided valuable insight that helped in care coordination so healthcare providers could provide timely and appropriate intervention and avoid unnecessary readmissions. Insight into patients' perceived gains in their understanding of health information can assist providers in meeting patients' resource needs and improve patient outcomes.

Summary

- As healthcare becomes more patient oriented, providers must treat each patient as an individual. The aspiration of a new patient-oriented community of care can only become reality by addressing each patient's health literacy needs.

■ The medagogy framework offers a pathway for educating individuals and can be beneficial in management of chronic illness. Treatment and management of chronic illness translates financially into more than $1 trillion dollars of the annual federal healthcare budget.

■ Patient education should include evaluative techniques to assess patient understanding. Historically, standard knowledge measurement that is traditional to academic settings has not been used in healthcare.

■ Universally, health literacy definitions acknowledge patients' needs to understand and utilize health information to which they have been exposed. Feldman and McPhee (2008) acknowledge that comprehension and understanding are abstract; therefore, direct measurement is often challenging.

■ In healthcare, the patient's perception of his personal understanding of information offers the provider an opportunity to determine where the patient thinks his knowledge exists on some continuum. Insight into personal perceptions can help the healthcare provider determine what the patient has mastered as well as the areas of deficit. Based on this data, the healthcare provider can develop an intervention that is specific, targeted, and culturally relevant for the patient.

■ The Wong-Baker pain scale offers a proven and reliable patient perception tool to communicate patients' pain intensity.

■ The simple utility of the Wong-Baker scale, translated into a tool for patient communication of personal perception, could revolutionize patient education efforts.

■ The understanding personal perception (UPP) scale offers an alternative method of communicating with patients regarding their level or depth of understanding about particular phenomena related to their health status. It shares the visual feature with a Likert scale measurement that is evident in the Wong-Baker scale.

■ The UPP tool was designed using a sun and clouds to represent clarity and clearness, or fuzziness and confusion of information, and depth of understanding about the topic being discussed.

■ The sun and cloud images are fashioned in a stair-step manner that is symbolic of upward progression, indicating personal understanding and a sense of self-efficacy. Each step is a numbered point on the five-point Likert scale.

■ The UPP tool strives to measure the two common themes consistently identified in health literacy: understanding and the ability to act.

- The tool uses two questions that the provider asks the patient:
  1. "How clear is your present understanding of this information, previously reviewed with or provided to you?" This lets providers know if they can build on present understanding or if they need to clear up any misunderstanding by focusing on areas where there is lack of clarity.
  2. "How comfortable are you with your understanding and ability to act on or carry out this information?" It is expected that a lack of understanding may influence patients' perceptions of their ability to act. Surprisingly, action is not always contingent on understanding, but action without understanding can pose safety risks.
- One of the challenges associated with health literacy is how best to communicate with patients and connect with their personal view within the context of improving health.
- The UPP tool provides unique insight into where patients envision their understanding and ability. Although the conception of the UPP tool originated in healthcare as a tool to be used between the patient and the provider, its use is not limited to the healthcare setting. Portability and ease of use make the tool attractive in any situation clear communication and understanding are needed.
- In the Centers for Medicare and Medicaid Services (CMS) care transitions pilot program, the UPP scale aided in transitioning patients into self-care safely and helped in care coordination so that healthcare providers intervened in a timely and appropriate way to avoid unnecessary readmissions.

Section IV Summary

Patient education empowers the patient with health autonomy through personal health knowledge. The process of patients arriving at their healthcare decisions, according to medagogy, is intimately connected to patient health knowledge, individualism, and the weight of external and internal influences. The patient education model, PITS, offers a pathway for healthcare providers to use when educating patients. Medagogy offers an overarching framework for patient education conceptual structures. Medagogy offers insight into an unprecedented theoretical view of patient internalization of information as the patient maneuvers through influences and generates personal healthcare decisions.

Whereas health literacy aims to identify patient deficits in the knowledge of health, medagogy focuses on the method by which patient individualism is central to patient understanding in the education process, thus promoting patient literacy. Medagogy focuses on providers meeting patients at the patients' level of health knowledge, and transitioning the interaction to patient-centered information exchange. The UPP scale allows the healthcare provider to gain insight into patients' perceptions and comfort with their ability to act upon information. Tools found in the research literature are long, cumbersome, not well used in the healthcare setting, and are disease-rather than patient-focused.

The simplicity of the Wong-Baker pain scale along with its ability to capture patients' perception provided the impetus for the UPP scale. The UPP scale uses pictures of clouds and the sun to signify clarity of understanding.

Although an abundance of data regarding health literacy and patient education can be found in the literature, standard universal strategic patient education delivery remains inconsistent at the point of service in daily practice. Illumination of the profundity of this healthcare problem should inspire the need for immediate action to progress patient knowledge as the result of patient-centered education via established patient-provider partnership. Peer interpretation is encouraged and welcomed as the role of the patient educator evolves through evidence-based practice. No two patients are exactly the same, and no two patient educational sessions should be identical.

Author's Final Thoughts

We can no longer just treat; we must teach and reach every patient. Through understanding our patients as individuals, we can give them a sense of personal priority and health direction. Prescriptive precedence is an exercise in futility. Only through shared knowledge and partnership in healthcare decision making can optimal healthcare outcomes be attained. PITS © and WHO allows patients to see "behind the curtain" by exposing them to expert knowledge that drives healthcare decisions. The informational seasons, hierarchy of patient education, medagogy conceptual framework, and UPP scale all serve to help the provider center information around the patient and their goals rather than around the elusive concept of health.

CHAPTER 13

Partnership: The NEW Model of Healthcare

Healthcare evolved from a desire to help the sick and infirmed. Many hospitals and centers for care originated as a form of ministry outreach by leaders and members of the church. In that original model the onus of care was on the healthcare provider to identify the problem, plan a course of care, identify appropriate therapies for healing, and follow-up as the provider deemed necessary. As providers in the 21st Century, the paradigm of healthcare is shifting. Healthcare is a career, one that can yield mighty salaries and although providers still plan healthcare treatment, the need for the role of the patient to transform from passive participant to active partner has never been needed more. Healthcare costs continue to soar and people are now surviving horrific accidents and injuries. People with chronic illnesses live longer. Medical miracles are happening every day. As people who benefit from these miracles live longer, many often live sicker, and the cost of care continues to soar. No longer can the healthcare field absorb all the responsibility for patient care. The time has arrived when consumers of healthcare can longer be bystanders in their own healthcare. Healthcare consumers must become active and knowledgeable in their healthcare. "Activated" consumers have been shown to decrease the fiscal burden associated with healthcare services (Colombara et al., 2015).

Healthcare has come a long way from the one room with multiple patient beds to patient rooms that look like hotel suites. In today's thriving healthcare business, healthcare institutions advertise from billboards to commercials, reminding consumers of their services and how much they care about them. Instead of waiting for patients to seek services, providers are inviting prospective patients to come see them for services. Many providers reach into the community through health fairs and public events offering information on prevention and/or early intervention, which may offset potential complications that could be associated with lifestyle, aging, or genetics.

The New Paradigm of Healthcare

Instead of using the traditional term healthcare, in which consumers act because of a change in their health, maybe today's new paradigm of healthcare delivery should be inverted to read as "care health," because today, prevention is the focus of healthcare. Today, the healthcare field is begging consumers to partner and become accountable in their health, while providers strive to offset negative health issues noted on the consumer's present path. Unfortunately, warnings and guidance concerning the negative impact of health behavior are often ignored and rarely followed.

For change to occur there must be action and buy in from the patient. Patients need to determine their goals and their path for health. It is at this point healthcare becomes an archaic term that should be replaced with a more accurate term like *patient-centered care* that defines the one in control as the center of power. Although patient-centered care has been a term associated with quality care in today's world, it is really more of a power shift where the power of choice and decision lies with the receiver of services, the patient. Some may argue that person-centered care should be the term of choice; however, there is still a level of dependence and vulnerability associated with the term, patient, that helps to remind the provider of the need to recognize the patient's lack of understanding of healthcare terminology and their dependence on the provider for improved health outcomes.

Patient-Centered Care Involves Activation

For healthcare interventions to be effective and last beyond one office visit, the patient and/or receiver of healthcare services must at some point activate. Activation as defined by the Merriam-Webster dictionary (2018) is derived from the core word, active; as to become active, to start working, or to cause to start working.

Optimal outcomes in care today and in the future are not just based on improvement in health. Optimal outcomes include a patient who is knowledgeable about their personal health, and knows how to care for self from acute and chronic health insults. Ideally, the patient is knowledgeable enough to detect changes in their body, such as alterations noted from disease, aging, or overall health changes. This does not lessen the provider's role; instead it helps to broaden it. The provider is more than a diagnosis and treatment source; they are also an educator and partner. The provider serves as the expert of health and the patient is the expert of self. They are both teachers and learners as they constantly exchange information from their area of expertise.

The PITS model as discussed earlier in Chapter 10 serves as a common pathway for information delivery, allowing providers to deliver information according to brain-based teaching methodology. When coupled with the understanding personal perception (UPP) tool (Chapter 12), the provider knows where the patient is in their learning progression, and can reinforce and intervene as needed to prevent negative outcomes such as readmission or error. The only down side to the PITS model is if the provider does not deliver the information or the patient doesn't realize the provider is delivering relevant information, therefore missing the possible learning that could have occurred in that teachable moment.

To help ensure the patient receives the information needed to be an active partner in their care, the WHY self-activation model was created. Similar to the PITS model, the WHY self-activation model serves to provide the patient with the information needed to make conscious decisions about their care and ultimately aids the patient in carrying out their goals for health.

Through visual cuing or knowledge of the WHY model, the healthcare consumer can initiate the information gathering process from the provider. Through use of the WHY model, the healthcare consumer will be able to obtain the information they will need to make personal healthcare choices. The healthcare consumer should also be able to understand WHY they are being asked to take medication and make any behavior or lifestyle changes. Most of all, the patient should be able to determine whether or not they agree with the provider's diagnosis and/or treatment plan. If the healthcare consumer is lost or cannot relate to the information, then patient activation or treatment compliance will not be likely. Instead of noncompliance being something the provider finds out about after discharge or the visit, the WHY model exposes all areas of treatment the patient needs to know. This exposure allows the patient to question, discuss, and refute the contingent plan, which in turn offers the provider a chance to personalize the treatment plan to one that is most suitable for the patient's life. It is at this point you can see where the patient is no longer a passenger in their care, but instead they are a partner. Whether the patient speaks up or not, that WHY model offers full disclosure for treatment choices therefore shifting the onus of care and ultimately health on to the owner, the patient. Any breach or change in the treatment plan by the patient should be communicated to the provider so that the patient's plan of care can stay up to date.

Alteration in the care plan should not be assumed to be an act of noncompliance, but instead it should be seen as personalization, as the patient tries to adapt their healthcare treatment plan into their daily life. It is important that the personalization of the treatment plan is safe and effective. The active transitioning of normal life and/or personal routines displays the patient's acceptance of the proposed diagnosis. The patient's personal commitment to their treatment plan can be further noted through active personal change in response to the healthcare provider's advice. This personal effort and adjustment reveals a patient commitment to comply with treatment. This commitment is important as the patient carries out the 3As of an activated patient: acceptance, action, and alteration. It is also important that the healthcare provider provides the patient with realistic timelines and follow-up, as well as treatment and follow-up outcomes and expectations. This will allow the patient to gauge progress or setback. In addition, the patient knows how they can intervene early to decrease avoidable damage and unnecessary costs.

As mentioned earlier, the WHY self-activation model mirrors the PITS model; Figure 13.1 displays how the steps of PITS merge with the WHY model and demonstrates how the WHY patient activation model consists of three steps. The first step is "W: what is wrong?" In the W step, the patient is exposed to the pathophysiology of the diagnosis, disease, injury, or ailment. In this stage, the provider shares the name of the condition, illness, or diagnosis. While the provider is discussing their assessment findings and medical opinion regarding the diagnosis, it helps to have visuals to use to assist the patient in seeing what the provider is discussing or referencing. The goal of the W stage of WHY is to begin to lay a stable foundation of understanding of the diagnosis so that as the provider moves forward, the patient can move toward the 3As of an activated patient: acceptance, action, and alteration.

In "H: how do you know?" the provider explains the symptomology associated with the diagnosed condition. Progress in condition is usually associated with progression of disease or physical aliment. It is in this stage the patient should be able to see their presenting signs and symptoms and/or be exposed to what may happen regarding symptoms, if not treated. The more symptomology noted in the patient's assessment, the more the patient will be able to identify the proposed health condition.

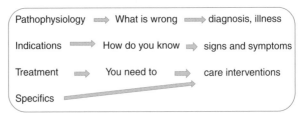

Fig. 13.1   PITS model symmetry with WHY patient activation model. © Melissa N. Stewart.

Lastly, the stage of the WHY model is "Y: you need to." This stage of the model is where the change in behavior occurs. It is in this stage that the provider ties the physical findings from W, to the presenting symptomology of H, to the requested action, and/or behavior changes of Y. This final stage is built on the rationale from the assessment findings and disclosed symptomology. This is the stage where the patient must act. This is when the patient must assume responsibility and become an active partner in their care. If the patient fits some or part of the advised course of treatment into their life, then they are making an active choice. If there is no adoption of advised treatment, then another walk through the WHY model may help open dialogue between patient and provider. Patients may not see themselves in the description of the disease and the symptoms; if that is the case, then patients may be in denial and or they may believe it is something else. Either way, there needs to be further discussion between the patient and the provider. Without discussion and/or clarity, action may not happen and/or it may not be the right action for that patient.

Knowing that providers who diagnose may not have time to sit down and gather all of the needed information, it is reasonable to assume another colleague could sit down and have the patient walk them through WHY from the patient's perspective. What do you think is wrong? How do you know this…signs and symptoms? You feel you need change or to do what to get better?

Know Your WHY - Patient Self Activation Model

What do you think is wrong?
How do you know this…signs and symptoms?
You feel you need change or to do what to get better?

© Melissa N. Stewart.

EXAMPLE OF THE WHY MODEL IN USE

Brandon is a 35-year-old male who is suffering from headaches. Brandon has made an appointment with Dr. Gautreaux today to find out what is wrong. After collecting Brandon's medical history and completing his physical exam, Dr. Gautreaux sits down to talk with him. Suddenly, nurse Michaelyn enters the room to consult with Dr. Gautreaux about another patient. After nurse Michaelyn exits, Dr. Gautreaux turns back to Brandon to discuss her findings. Dr. Gautreaux shares that Brandon appears to be suffering from hypertension, better known as high blood pressure. Brandon stops Dr. Gautreaux and says questioningly, "that doesn't seem right, I'm having headaches not chest pain." Dr. Gautreaux answers, "let's look at why."

> W: what is wrong. Hypertension occurs when the force of blood flow inside the arteries is elevated. When hypertension occurs, your heart has to work harder to get blood out to reoxygenate your body.

> H: signs and symptoms. Your blood pressure today was 184/106. Ideal blood pressure for a man your age is top number 120 to 129 and bottom number 80 or less. You stated you had a light headache.

> Y: you need to. Decrease your salt intake. All of that fast food you mentioned in your history is not good for your arteries. Also, work on controlling your stress. You mentioned that your job has been extremely stressful. Try to sneak some joy and relaxation into your work environment. I am also going to start you on Lasix, 25 mg every morning. The Lasix is to help you get rid of that extra fluid you mentioned, swollen hands and feet. Let's do this for 2 months, then I would like to see you again. How does that sound to you Brandon?

After Dr. Gautreaux finished reviewing Brandon's diagnosis using the WHY model, Brandon answered the doctor with, "I think I can do that," and a smile.

Patient education does not have to be wordy and intimidating. In fact, the simpler it is, the easier it is received. The WHY model offers a simple pathway for health information delivery. The pathway can be initiated by the patient and or the provider. For example, Dr. Gautreaux could have forgotten where she was in the course of the visit when she was disturbed by her nurse and then forgotten to initiate WHY. If this would have occurred, then Brandon could have simply asked Dr. Gautreaux about the poster in her waiting room and in the examination room that says Ask Your Provider WHY. This would have triggered provider use of the WHY model. Either way, Brandon leaves knowing why and is empowered to make an informed decision regarding his participation in his care. According to Colombara et al. (2015) and Akoko et al. (2017), knowing why you are asked to do something can increase the likelihood of compliance.

Author's Final Words

We can no longer just treat, we must teach and reach every patient. Through patient understanding, personal priority and health direction can be gained. Prescriptive precedence is an exercise in futility. Only through shared knowledge and partnership in health decisions can optimal healthcare outcomes be attained. The PITS and WHY patient education delivery models allow the patient to see behind the curtain by exposing them to rationale for behavior change and expert knowledge that drives healthcare decisions. The informational seasons, hierarchy of patient education, medagogy conceptual framework, and UPP tool all serve to help the provider center information around patient instead of around the elusive concept of health.

CHAPTER 14

Legal Implications Associated With Patient Education

Dawn Morris

The failure to assess a patient's level of health literacy during care or treatment may subject a healthcare provider to legal action. Patient education is essential, and failure to properly provide such education may constitute a breach of a legal or ethical duty. However, such education must be appropriated to the patient, under a patient-centered needed model, each patient's level of literacy must be assessed to ensure that health education is being provided at an appropriate, comprehensible level for each patient.

Healthcare providers must understand that a patient's level of educational attainment does not necessarily equate to a patient's health literacy level or level of understanding. For example, according to the 2003 National Assessment of Adult Literacy, only 30% of individuals with a Bachelor's degree or higher are proficient in health literacy (Kutner, 2006). In addition, physicians and nurses often overestimate a patient's health literacy (Kelly and Haidet, 2007; Dickens et al., 2013).

Where a duty exists between a healthcare provider and a patient, the healthcare provider owes an obligation to act according to the applicable standards of care, and a failure to do so can result in negligence of malpractice. The duty to educate patients about their disease processes and treatment regimen is one owed by healthcare providers, but simply handing a patient preprepared educational material without assessing the patient' ability to understand such material may well constitute a breach of the duty owed, subjecting the healthcare provider to potential liability.

Law Versus Ethics

A key factor in determining whether a legal obligation exists to assess an individual's level of health literacy is whether there is a duty to do so. Duties arise from many sources, but the deeply entrenched bases are found in law and ethics, similar but distinct concepts.

ETHICS

At its simplest, ethics refers to what is right or wrong. Ethics is an area of philosophy that examines conduct, moral judgment, and the way values influence choices. Rules of ethics guide moral choices and address moral dilemmas that arise during healthcare relationships (Dewey et al., 2018). Healthcare ethics, or bioethics, is a specific field of study that addresses issues of life and death, basic human rights, such as autonomy and dignity, and the rights of individuals with disabilities. Ethical or moral decisions are inherent in healthcare, and healthcare providers are faced with ethical dilemmas and decisions on a daily or near-daily basis. In healthcare settings, healthcare providers' decisions are influenced by ethical principles in the way they provide care to and make decisions about patients. Certain basic principles of ethics help define essential ethical obligations, and these principles should not be violated absent compelling reasons to override them (Chulay and Burns, 2010). Some of these fundamental principles of ethics include autonomy, beneficence, nonmaleficence, justice, and veracity (Chulay and Burns, 2010). Autonomy is that which regards a person's right to make decisions for themselves based on their personal values and beliefs and includes, for example, the capacity to make decisions and the ability to make informed consent without coercion. Beneficence is the obligation to prevent harm while doing good. On the other hand, nonmaleficence refers to the principle of "do no harm" and includes the obligation of a healthcare provider to maintain professional competence and to practice within the scope of practice and applicable standards of care. Justice includes ensuring equal access and equitable distribution of resources. Veracity refers to the truthfulness of communications between the healthcare provider and the patient.

Dr. Smith Helps Pregnant Ann with Equal Access to Resources She can Understand

Dr. Smith works a shift at an urban health care clinic. He is asked to see Ann, an 18-year old female, who is pregnant. Ann has received no prenatal care because she is uninsured and is homeless because her parents kicked her out of her home on learning of her pregnancy. Ann is a senior in high school and will graduate with her class next month, but she acknowledges that she has struggled academically and, because of her current homelessness, has missed a lot of classes. Ann wants to keep her baby but expresses concern about her ability to do so.

Dr. Smith, in obtaining Ann's history, recognizes Ann's autonomy to make the decision about whether or not to keep her baby. Under the principles of beneficence and justice, Dr. Smith recognizes that Ann is in need of community resources and does not have the knowledge needed to access these resources.

Dr. Smith arranges for Ann to talk to a clinic social worker and case manager regarding Ann's current state of homelessness and lack of insurance. Dr. Smith also arranges for Ann to be seen by an OB-GYN. Dr. Smith acknowledges that based on her history, although Ann has almost graduated from high school, her health literacy may not be equivalent to her educational attainment level, so before providing any education or discussing medical diagnoses and treatment, Dr. Smith assesses Ann's health literacy level. This demonstrates nonmaleficence in that Dr. Smith did not simply hand Ann copies of available educational material but determined that Ann likely needed some alternative teaching methods to understand the relevant issues fully. Finally, Dr. Smith showed respect to Ann throughout his assessment and treatment and was honest in informing her of the potential risks of lack of prenatal treatment to both her and the baby.

Law

Black's Law Dictionary defines law as "a body of rules of action or conduct prescribed by controlling authority and having binding legal force" (Black's Law Dictionary, 1990). The failure to obey or comply with laws may subject one to civil or criminal sanctions or legal consequences. Claims of professional malpractice or negligence arise under laws enacted by the individual state or under federal laws. There are several types of laws that apply or may apply to healthcare providers. These include constitutional law, administrative law, criminal law, contract law, and tort law. Administrative laws include state or federal agencies, such as state medical or nursing boards that govern those professions. Criminal law applies when actions rise to the level of criminal action, such as assault and battery. Tort, or civil, law concerns reparations for damages resulting from negligence.

Difference Between Malpractice and Negligence

Although the terms "malpractice" and "negligence" are sometimes used interchangeably, they are two different things. Negligence is a broader legal concept that applies to anyone, whereas malpractice is limited to those whose actions arise under a professional license. Negligence is harm caused by a breach of a duty but malpractice, on the other hand, means that a licensed healthcare provider failed to meet professional standards in the treatment of a patient. Both negligence and malpractice may result in harm or damages to a patient, but malpractice is about violating professional standards, and negligence is a failure to act in a reasonably prudent manner. Although malpractice requires the existence of a relationship between the professional and the harmed individual, no such relationship is required for negligence to occur.

MALPRACTICE

Malpractice is professional misconduct that includes, for example, an unreasonable lack of professional skill, the failure to meet professional standards of care, or the improper discharge of professional duties. Malpractice occurs when the individual rendering professional services fails to exercise that degree of skill and competence of an average, prudent, and reputable member of the profession and which skill is expected under all the circumstances in a given locality that results in injury, loss, or damage to the patient (Black's Law Dictionary, 1990).

The concept of malpractice applies to those healthcare providers who are required by law to be licensed to practice. A license is a permit granted by a governmental body or agency to an individual, firm, or corporation that allows them to function in a profession, such as law, medicine, and nursing, subject to regulation (Black's Law Dictionary, 1990). Professional licensure permits a qualified individual to perform designated skills and service in a given jurisdiction. For many professions, licensure is mandatory, and engagement in the profession without a valid license is illegal. For example, practicing medicine or nursing without a valid license is subject to criminal and civil sanctions. Those who do hold a valid professional license are subject to regulations and are required to operate within the applicable scope of practice and the licensing statute.

NEGLIGENCE

Negligence is "conduct that falls below the standard established by law for the protection of others against unreasonable risks of harm" (Black's Law Dictionary, 1990). Negligence may occur by an affirmative act that falls below applicable standards, but it can also occur because of an omission to act. An omission may be an intentional or unintentional failure to act. Essential to a negligence claim is the existence of a duty, breach of that duty, and harm or damages caused by that breach (Table 14.1).

Acts of negligence or malpractice are torts, although some may rise to the level of criminal action. Tort claims flow throw the civil court system. The purpose of tort law is to make the injured party whole again, primarily through monetary compensation or damages. Torts may be intentional or unintentional. An intentional tort is an intentional act that violates another person's rights or property. Intentional acts may also rise to the level of or be considered as criminal offenses. Criminal negligence occurs when acts are grossly or wantonly negligent. Assault, battery, and false imprisonment

TABLE 14.1 ▧ **Definitions of Negligence Elements**

Element of Negligence	Definition
Duty	An obligation to conform to legal standard of reasonable conduct in light of apparent risk
Breach	The breaking or violation of a law, right, obligation, engagement or duty, either through commission or omission
Causation	The fact of being the cause of something produced or of happening; the act whereby an effect is produced *Proximate cause:* substantial factor in bringing about harm; but for causation (but for event A, event B would not have occurred) *Cause-in-fact:* that particular cause that produces an event and without which the event would not have occurred
Harm, damages	*Harm:* the existence of loss or detriment in fact of any kind to a person resulting from any cause *Damage:* loss, injury, or deterioration caused by the negligence, design, or accident of one person to another, in respect of the latter's person or property

Black's Law Dictionary, 6th ed. 1990. St. Paul, MN, West Publishing.

are examples of actions that may be considered as either or both torts and crimes. An unintentional tort is an unintended wrongful act against another that produces injury or harm; it is this that is commonly understood to be negligence.

Negligence, Not Malpractice

Mr. Carte, a resident in a nursing home, fell while being transferred from a toilet to his bed. He later died as a result of his injuries. An appellate court in Ohio ruled that the lawsuit was one for common law negligence and not malpractice because the fall did not result while going to or coming from medical treatment or diagnosis, but was simply a case of Mr. Carte using the restroom (*Carte v. Manor of Whitehall*, 2014 Ohio 5670; Ohio App. 2014).

Malpractice

Ms. Hamilton, a resident in a nursing home, died following complications from a fractured femur. There was no indication that a fall occurred, but the court found that the nursing home's failure to discover and failure to diagnose the fractured femur constituted negligence in failing to provide appropriate medical treatment and services (*Hamilton v. Baton Rouge Health Care*, 52 So. 3d 330; La. App. 2010).

Assault and Battery

Joshua, a minor, was admitted to the hospital following an accidental overdose of prescribed medications. At midnight, Joshua was ambulating in his assigned room when several hospital staff attempted to force Joshua back into bed. Joshua and his mother filed claims for assault and battery. The court found that the entire record demonstrated that Hopebridge was a healthcare provider; because the alleged assault and battery occurred while Hopebridge was providing medical care, or healthcare, or patient safety, the claims against Hopebridge were presumptively healthcare liability claims. The claim was dismissed, however, on technical procedural issues for failure to file an expert report in a timely fashion under applicable Texas law (*Hopebridge Hosp. Hous., L.L.C. v. Lerma, 521 S.W.3d 830*; Tex. App., 2017.)

Duties

REQUISITE PATIENT–HEALTHCARE PROVIDER RELATIONSHIP

A healthcare provider does not owe a legal duty to a patient unless a professional relationship exists between them. Such a professional relationship essentially forms a contract between the patient and healthcare professional. In such a relationship, the provider owes duties of professional competence and compliance with the applicable standards or care, and the patient owes duties of adherence to recommended treatment and truthfulness. Generally, a physician-patient relationship commences when a physician agrees to or takes affirmative action to diagnose or treat a patient with the patient's implied or express consent. When a physician treats an unconscious patient in the emergency room, the patient has not expressly consented to treatment, but consent in that situation is implied (Schwab, 2007). This is a mutual consensual relationship with the patient knowingly seeking physician services and the physician knowingly accepting the patient. Once this relationship forms, legal obligations and duties are imposed on the physician. Physician-patient relationships generally do not arise from the making of an initial appointment or from informal opinions (e.g., curbside consultations) given to a colleague regarding patient care, although courts in some circumstances have found such relationships (Schwab, 2007). For example, if a physician offers professional advice to an individual while both attend a party, a relationship sufficient to impose legal duties may arise if the healthcare provider intended the individual to rely on the advice, and the individual did so to his detriment.

A professional relationship must also exist between nonphysician, professional healthcare providers before the imposition of legal duties. For example, nurses' duties to patients arise when a nurse-patient relationship is formed.

This generally occurs during a nurse's scope of employment when the nurse accepts a patient assignment and ends when another nurse takes over responsibility for the patient. A nurse-patient relationship may also develop outside the scope of employment when a nurse voluntarily forms such a relationship through the provision of nursing services. Many states have "Good Samaritan" laws, which provide some protection against legal claims when a healthcare provider stops to render aid in an emergency, but violations of professional standards of care in such situations could still give rise to legal liability.

Provider-Patient Relationship

A young child exhibited new symptomology, possibly indicating a malfunction of a ventriculoperitoneal shunt. During the course of attempting to evaluate and diagnose the new symptomology, her pediatrician consulted with a pediatric intensivist, Dr. Smith, at another hospital. Dr. Smith subsequently telephoned Dr. Gilmartin, a pediatric neurologist, and discussed the child's symptoms and whether or not a surgery was indicated. Dr. Gilmartin never saw the child or spoke to the child's parents. The child suffered severe brain damage before the surgery could be performed. The court dismissed the lawsuit against Dr. Gilmartin, finding that there was no patient-physician relationship between him and the child because where a physician gives an "informal opinion," at the request of a treating physician, and owes no duty to the patient because no physician-patient relationship is created (*Irvin v. Smith*, 31 P.3d 934, 272 Kan. 112; Kan., 2001).

Good Samaritan Laws

A nurse hired as an independent contractor by a school was to be available to render aid to students; however, at the site of the field trip, the nurse rendered aid to a child who was not a member of the school. The nonstudent child injured his eye and, because of infection and complications, later lost his eye. The court determined that the nurse was immune from liability under the state's Good Samaritan law (*McDaniel v. Keck*, 53 A.D.3d 869, 861 N.Y.S.2d 516, 2008 NY Slip Op 6321; N.Y. App. Div., 2008).

SOURCES OF DUTIES FOR HEALTHCARE PROFESSIONALS

An essential element in a claim of negligence or malpractice is the existence of a duty owed by a healthcare provider to the patient. Such duties arise from many sources and will often be evaluated by a court on a case by case basis. Such duties or obligations may arise from law, scope of professional practice, and standards of care, among others.

Scope of Practice Versus Standards of Care

Scope of Practice. Scope of practice is defined by state law and refers to the professional activities defined under state law. For example, the scope of practice for registered nurses is set forth in nurse practice acts as adopted by each state's legislature. A scope of practice act sets forth the minimum required education, experience, and professional competencies and sets forth those professional activities that a healthcare provider is permitted to undertake under the terms of his or her professional licensure. Professional boards, such as boards of medicine or boards of nursing, are established under professional practice acts, and these boards are authorized to enforce and administer the rules and regulations established by the acts. For example, state boards of medicine regulate the practice of medicine, including licensure, discipline, investigation, and certification of its members. In many states, the board of medicine also oversees and regulates many other healthcare professions including, for example, physicians' assistants, respiratory therapists, and radiology technicians.

Standards of Care. Standards of care are defined from healthcare and legal perspectives, both of which can be relied on when determining whether a professional duty is owed to a patient in any given circumstance. In healthcare, a standard of care is the process that a healthcare provider should follow for a certain type of patient, illness, or clinical circumstance when diagnosing or treating a patient (Shiel, n.d.). For example, the American Diabetes Association maintains standards of medical care in diabetes and the American Association of Critical Care Nurses sets forth standards of care for critical care nurses.

On the other hand, standard of care from a legal perspective refers to the way similarly qualified healthcare providers would have acted under the same or similar circumstances (Shiel, n.d.). The standard of care is a legal measure in malpractice or negligence cases to determine whether the healthcare provider's alleged wrongful conduct was an act performed or omitted that an ordinary, reasonably prudent provider, in the same or similar circumstances, would have done or not done.

Under both perspectives, however, standards of care refer to the minimum criteria for a healthcare professionals' competency or proficiency and establish criteria that serve as a basis of comparison when evaluating the quality of healthcare. In essence, standards of care define quality care and provide specific criteria that can be used to determine if quality of care has been provided (Gura, 2004). Failure to follow standards of care, such as the standards of nursing practice set forth by the American Nurses' Association, may result in negligence or malpractice.

Other Sources of Standards of Care

Institutional Policies. Duties may also arise from policies adopted by healthcare organizations. In negligence or malpractice cases, healthcare providers' actions are judged by the applicable standard of care or what is reasonably prudent care under the circumstances. However, situations may occur where the standard of care is met, but a hospital policy has been violated, and this can result in a claim of negligence or substandard care.

Institutions adopt policies for purposes of providing safety and high-quality care to patients and to prevent liability. Policies serve many purposes, such as facilitating compliance with standards of care and reducing variation from these standards. Institutional policies also promote compliance with various regulations, statutes, and accreditation requirements such as HIPAA (Health Insurance Portability and Accountability Act of 1996) privacy rules and Joint Commission accreditation requirements.

In some cases, however, policies may be inconsistent with applicable standards of care, professional practice guidelines, or laws, and these inconsistencies can result in claims of negligence or malpractice. For example, although policies are generally considered to be guidelines rather than mandates, policies that are inflexible or that eliminate clinical judgment or individualized care can lead to legal claims if a provider deviates even slightly from the policy, even though the care provided met the standard of care (Destache, 2013).

Evidence-Based Practice. Duties may also arise from evidenced-based practice. The most common definition of evidence-based practice (EBP) is from Sackett and colleagues. EBP is "the conscientious, explicit and judicious use of current best evidence in making decisions about the care of the individual patient. It means integrating individual clinical expertise with the best available external clinical evidence from systematic research" (Sacket et al., 1996). EBP is the integration of clinical expertise, patient values, and the best research evidence into the decision-making process for patient care, where clinical expertise refers to the clinician's cumulated experience, education, and clinical skills. (Sackett et al., 1996). Evidence-based standards of care must rest on the best available evidence that emerges from a concerted hypothesis-driven process of research synthesis and meta-analysis (Barkhordarian et al., 2011).

The Institute of Medicine (IOM) is a nonprofit organization that is a component of the US National Academy of Science. IOM provides guidance on issues related to health and medicine and also provides evidence-based research and recommendations for health policy. The IOM has set forth several core competencies for healthcare workers, one of which is the use of EBP through integration of best research with clinical expertise and patient values to provide optimum care (Table 14.2; IOM, 2003).

Scientific evidence should be considered when developing standards of care in implementing patient-centered interventions. Patient-centered standards of care include consideration of a patient's gender, ethnicity, health history, socioeconomic status, and many other factors, including the best available research evidence. This affects how standards are established for clinical decision making and optimal patient outcomes. (Barkhordarian et al., 2011).

TABLE 14.2 ■ **Institute of Medicine Core Competencies for Health Care Workers**

Core Competency	Description
Provide patient-centered care	Identify, respect, and care about patients' differences, values, preferences, and expressed needs; relieve pain and suffering. Coordinate continuous care; listen to, clearly inform, communicate with, and educate patients. Share decision making and management. Continuously advocate disease prevention, wellness, and promotion of healthy lifestyles, including a focus on population health.
Work in interdisciplinary teams	Cooperate, collaborate, communicate, and integrate care in teams to ensure that care is continuous and reliable.
Employ evidence-based practice	Integrate best research with clinical expertise and patient values for optimum care, and participate in learning and research activities to the extent feasible.
Apply quality improvement	Identify errors and hazards in care. Understand and implement basic safety design principles, such as standardization and simplification. Continually understand and measure quality of care in terms of structure, process, and outcomes in relation to patient and community needs. Design and test interventions to change processes and systems of care, with the objective of improving quality.
Use informatics	Communicate, manage knowledge, mitigate error, and support decision making using information technology.

IOM, Institute of Medicine Committee on the Health Professions Education Summit (2003). Greiner AC, Knebel E, editors. *Health Professions Education: A Bridge to Quality.* Washington, DC: National Academies Press. Available at: https://www.ncbi.nlm.nih.gov/books/NBK221528.

Codes of Ethics. Professional codes of ethics, although not legally binding, may also contribute to duties owed by healthcare professionals to patients. Codes of ethics set forth fundamental values and commitments of healthcare professionals. For example, the Code of Ethics for Nurses with Interpretive Statements is a social contract between nurses and the public that "exemplifies the profession's promise to provide and advocate for safe quality care for all patients and communities" (American Nurses' Association [ANA], n.d.). The Code of Ethics for Nurses provides a statement of the profession's ethical values, obligations, and duties to those in the nursing profession and serves as a nonnegotiable ethical standard (ANA, n.d.). Likewise, the Principles of Medical Ethics are intended to address the elements of ethical behavior and, although they are not laws, they are standards of conduct for physicians (American Medical Association Council on Ethical and Judicial Affairs, n.d.; Riddick, 2003).

Many professional associations have adopted Codes of Ethics individualized to their professions. For example, the Coalition of National Health Education Organizations (CNHEO) has adopted a Code of Ethics (CNHEO, 2011), which states that:

> *The Code of Ethics provides a framework of shared values within the professions in which Health Education is practiced. The Code of Ethics is grounded in fundamental ethical principles including promoting justice, doing good, and avoidance of harm. The responsibility of each health educator is to aspire to the highest possible standards of conduct and to encourage the ethical behavior of all those with whom they work.*

Patient Bill of Rights. Duties may also be derived from the patient bills of rights. Many healthcare organizations and associations have adopted patient bills of rights. A bill of rights is a document that informs patients of goals and expectations for them during a course of medical treatment or hospitalization. These rights cover topics such as access to care, patient dignity, confidentiality, and consent. Although these bills of rights are generally not legally binding, their provisions may, nonetheless, give rise to a duty owed by a healthcare provider to a patient. Many bills of rights adopt language or statements from codes of ethics, and some include matters that have been written into state or federal law, which, if violated, can give rise to legal claims.

The National Institutes of Health (NIH) Clinical Center, for example, has adopted a Clinical Center Patients' Bill of Rights. Several rights are described in plain language, including the rights "to receive complete information about diagnosis, treatment and prognosis from the physician, in terms that are easily understood" and "to receive information necessary for you to give informed consent before procedure or treatment, including a description of the procedure or treatment, any potential risks or benefits, the probable duration of any incapacitation, and any alternatives" (US Department of Health and Human Services, National Institutes of Health, n.d.). The failure, then, to provide such information to a study participant may constitute a breach of a duty imposed by this bill of rights. Furthermore, because a patient has a right to receive information "in terms that are easily understood," the failure to assess whether a particular patient has understood the terms because of low health literacy may also constitute a breach of a duty.

Custom and Locality. Duties may also arise from local customs or practices. This is generally known as the "locality rule." In legal cases, healthcare providers are judged by the standard of care in the locality where the alleged wrongful act or omission occurred. As a result of evidence-based standards of care, provision of healthcare by different types of providers is becoming more and more standardized. However, generally accepted practices in certain locales may differ or conflict with generally accepted practices and standards. Situations may occur where a healthcare provider follows an accepted standard of care but may be found to have breached a duty because such a standard of care differs from local practices (Lewis et al., 2007).

Duties and health literacy

There is no exact list of duties owed by healthcare providers to patients. A patient's ability, or capacity, however, to understand, comprehend, make decisions, or consent to or refuse treatment is an important factor. A healthcare provider's failure to make a determination of whether a patient has such ability or capacity may constitute a breach of a duty. Health care providers assess a patient's decision-making capacity to a degree for purposes of obtaining informed consent or to determine if a patient with possible cognitive issues is capable of making decisions. Medical decision-making capacity has four key elements: (1) ability to demonstrate understanding of the benefits and risks of, and the alternatives to, a proposed treatment or intervention (including no treatment); (2) ability to demonstrate appreciation of those benefits, risks, and alternatives; (3) ability to show reasoning in making a decision; and (4) ability to communicate their choice (Physician's Weekly, 2012). Healthcare providers, however, should expand this to include the assessment of the capacity to understand health information or, in other words, assess a patient's health literacy level. The failure of healthcare providers to determine a patient's health literacy level could result in breaches of duties to provide education to a patient about their diagnoses, treatment, or prognosis; lack of informed consent for lack of capacity to understand the consent; negligence in discharge planning and instructions; and incapacity of the patient to understand instructions for proper self-administration of medication, among others.

Although the following case studies do not involve issues of health literacy, it is apparent that in each of these scenarios, an individual with low health literacy might be at greater risk for harm because of a greater chance of lack of understanding and knowledge.

Failure to Obtain Informed Consent

The plaintiff, Wilson, suffered foot drop following a hip replacement as a result of damage to his sciatic nerve during surgery. Wilson filed suit against Dr. Schaefer for failure to inform Wilson of the risk of damage to his sciatic nerve and foot drop and, had he been informed of the risk, he would not have elected to do the surgery. The doctor argued that informed consent was given by the anesthesiologist who advised Wilson of the risk of paralysis from anesthesia. The court agreed with Wilson, finding that informed consent to the risks from anesthesia is different than informed consent to risks associated with the physical removal and replacement of a hip (*Wilson v. Schaefer*, 2014 IL App (4th) 131043-U; Ill. App., 2014).

Negligent Discharge Instructions

A young man suffered a head injury and was treated in the emergency room. After observing the patient for 6 to 8 hours, the man was discharged home with his father. The treating physicians gave oral discharge instructions to the patient about symptoms to watch for with head injuries and when to return to the hospital, but neither provided written instructions, nor did they give instructions to the man's caregiver (his father). In addition, the physicians declined to provide a copy of the hospital's standard printed head injury instructions because of a disagreement with the verbiage. The young man was discharged and subsequently died at home as the result of an intracranial bleed. The court found that the physicians breached a duty of care to the young man (*Smith v. Univ. of Cincinnati*, 2012 Ohio 3646; Ohio Ct. Cl., 2012).

The Understanding Personal Perception Tool Pilot

Annette Knobloch

Psychometric properties of Stewart's Understanding Personal Perception (UPP) scale were tested with a small sample ($n = 15$) of nurse educators in conjunction with a continuing education session, "You and the Registry of Nursing Research Database, Virginia Henderson International Nursing Library, Sigma Theta Tau International." The study was approved by the Our Lady of the Lake College Institutional Review Board. Participants received a study packet consisting of pretest and posttest study forms, and the traditional Continuing Education Participant Evaluation form (CEPE; Our Lady of the Lake Health Career Institute). The forms in each packet were precoded with matching study numbers, which ensured anonymity while allowing the linkage of the three study forms to responders. Participation was optional, and completion of the forms constituted consent.

The pretest and posttest study forms consisted of the pictorial UPP rating scale placed horizontally below each of the six session objectives, such that there were six rows, each with a session objective and the UPP images. Stewart's UPP numeric ratings ranged from 1 to 5, with 1 representing the brightest sunshine image and 6 representing the darkest clouds. Therefore, lower scores indicated higher perceived understanding. The CEPE contained three sections:

- A block for rating the achievement of the same six session objectives, with a Likert scale worded Excellent, Good, Fair, Poor, n/a. Responses were coded 1, 2, 3, 4, respectively, and lower ratings indicated higher ratings. There were no participants who chose "n/a" (not applicable) responses.
- A block with the Likert scale ratings for the instructor's knowledge of content, presentation skills, and organization of content.

- A block with five overall program objectives related to the extent to which the session met expectations, the quality of the session and handouts, and the impact of the session on the participant. Three relevant subitems from the impact-related CEPE statement were treated as separate items in various analyses in this study: (1) increase your knowledge; (2) change a skill or attitude; and (c) change your practice performance.

The three study forms had high internal consistency values. Reliability and factor analyses (Table A.1) were performed for the pretest form, the posttest form, and the CEPE form, despite the small sample size for several reasons. First, conducting these analyses necessitated setting up data entry and data processing for potential use in future studies with larger samples and to provide results for this particular study. Second, there were no psychometric data available for the CEPE, and these analyses provided information for relevant sections of the CEPE for this study. Data from the six objective-related items in the first block and the three components of the impact-related statement were compiled and used for analyses in this study. Thus, CEPE items that were conceptually unrelated to the UPP were excluded, and the findings herein reported for the CEPE applied to the portions of the CEPE used in various study analyses. Despite the small sample size, principal component factor analysis, with varimax rotation, of the posttest UPP data supported construct validity; Kaiser-Meyer-Olkin (KMO) Measure of Sampling Adequacy (MSA) values, overall and per objective, were greater than .5, as were the communalities for each objective. A single factor emerged, with loadings ranging from .79 to .97.

A paired samples t-test revealed significantly higher ratings on the posttest, compared with the pretest, for each objective; for the set of objectives, t (14) ranged from 3.3 to 5.3, P ranged from < .001 to .005, and no confidence intervals for the mean difference contained 0. The P values were all less than .007, and thus were still significant at the overall .05 level after the Bonferroni adjustment for multiple comparisons. Higher posttest ratings provided additional support for construct validity for use of the UPP as a rating scale because it was expected that the participants' ratings for the session objectives would be higher after the session than before the session. The pretest and posttest study forms, using UPP as a rating scale in conjunction with the stated objectives, were able to detect differences in perceived understanding before and after the continuing education session.

The Pearson correlations between the UPP and CEPE ratings were not significant, ranging from –0.08 to 0.35, with P values ranging from .19 to .76.

TABLE A.1 ▨ Summary of Psychometric Properties for Forms in This Study; $n = 15$

Form	Items	Cronbach's Alpha	Factors	Range of Item Loadings on Factor	Factor Analysis			
					Variance Explained	KMO[a]	Range of MSA Values[a]	Range of Communalities
Pretest	6	0.98	One	0.89–0.98	90.4%	a	*	0.80–0.96
Posttest	6	0.95	One	0.79–0.97	82.6%	0.85	0.78–0.97	0.62–0.94
CEPE block I	6	0.98	One	0.91–0.97	91.5%	a	0.77–0.91	0.52–0.96
CEPE block I and impact items	9	0.91	Two	0.89–0.99 (objective items) 0.81–0.91 (impact items)	88.9%	a	a	0.84–0.97

[a] KMO (Kaiser-Meyer-Olkin) and MSA (measure of sampling adequacy) refer, respectively, to overall and individual item indices that aid in determining whether factor analysis is advisable.
[b] Undeterminable, probably because of very small sample size.

These nonsignificant correlations supported discriminate validity because the UPP measured perception of understanding related to the session objectives, but the CEPE measured achievement.

In summary, these findings demonstrate the effectiveness of the UPP rating scale for this study and provide support for additional testing of the tool with adequate sample sizes, various populations, and various research questions.

"Access". (2005). Access program reduces inappropriate admissions. *Hospital Case Management, 13*(5), 69–75.

"Activate". Merriam-Webster.com. Merriam-Webster, n.d. Web. 23 July 2018.

Ajzen, I., & Fishbein, M. (1980). *Understanding attitudes and predicting social behavior*. Englewood Cliffs, NJ: Prentice-Hall.

Akoko, B. M., Fon, P. N., Ngu, R. C., & Ngu, K. B. (2017). Knowledge of hypertension and compliance with therapy among hypertensive patients in the Bamenda health district of Cameroon: a cross-sectional study. *Cardiology and Therapy, 6*(1), 53–67.

Albert, N. M., Buchsbaum, R., & Li, J. (2007). Randomized study on the effect of video education on heart failure healthcare utilization, symptoms, and self-care behaviors. *Patient Education and Counseling, 69*(1), 129–139.

Albon, A. (2008). Reconstructing recall: room for improvement? Amanda Albon describes how psychologists have used knowledge about how memory works to improve the accuracy of eyewitness recall. *Psychology Review, 13*(3), 24–26.

Alexander, R. (2004). Still no pedagogy? Principle, pragmatism, and compliance in primary education. *Cambridge Journal of Education, 34*(1), 7–30.

Allen, R.M., & Jones, M. P. (1998). The validity and reliability for asthma knowledge questionnaire used in the evaluation of a group asthma self-management program for adults with asthma. *Journal of Asthma, 35*(7), 537–545.

American Hospital Association. (1973). *A patient's bill of rights*. Retrieved from http://www.patienttalk.info/AHA-Patient_Bill_of_Rights.htm.

American Medical Association Ad Hoc Committee on Health Literacy for the Council on Scientific Affairs. (1999). Health literacy: Report of the council of scientific affairs. *Journal of the American Medical Association, 281*(6), 552–557.

American Medical Association Council on Ethical and Judicial Affairs (CEJA). *Code of Medical Ethics* Available at: https://www.ama-assn.org/councils/council-ethical-judicial-affairs/about-council-ethical-judicial-affairs-ceja.

American Nurses' Association. *Code of Ethics for Nurses*. Available at: https://www.nursingworld.org/practice-policy/nursing-excellence/ethics/code-of-ethics-for-nurses.

American Nurses Association. (2004). *Nursing: Scope and standards of practice*. Washington, DC: Nursesbooks.org.

Anderson, J. G., Rainey, M. R., & Eysenbach, G. (2004). The impact of cyberhealth on the physician-patient relationship. *Journal of Medical Systems, 27*(1), 67–84.

Anderson, L. W., Krathwohl, D. R., Airsian, P. W., et al. (Eds.).(2001). *A taxonomy for learning, teaching, and assessment: A revision of Bloom's taxonomy of educational objectives*. New York: Longman.

Anderson, R. C., & Speiro, R. J. (1977). *Schooling and the acquisition of knowledge*. Hillsdale, NJ: Erlbaum.

Anderson, R. C., Spiro, R. J., & Montague, W. W. (Eds.), (1984). *Schooling and the acquisition of knowledge.* Hillsdale, NJ: Erlbaum.

Anonymous. (2009, September). Matching teaching strategies with adult learning styles maximizes education effectiveness. *Strategies for Nurse Managers, 9*(9), 7–9.

Aristotle. (2009). *Metaphysics.* (W.D. Ross, Trans.) U.S.: Classics-Unbound.

Atherton, J. S. (2009). *Learning and teaching: Misrepresentation, myths and misleading ideas.* Retrieved from http://www.learningandteaching.info/learning/myths.htm.

Ausubel, D. P., Novak, J. D., & Hanesian, H. (1986). *Educational psychology: A cognitive view* (2nd ed.). New York, NY: Werbel & Peck.

Avillion, A. E. (2009, October). Tailor education to appeal to all adult learning styles. *HCPro's Advisor to the ANCC Magnet Recognition Program, 5*(10), 6.

Avillion, A. E. (2009). *Learning styles in nursing education: Integrating teaching strategies into staff development.* Marblehead, MA: HCPro.

Bacon, F. (1893). *The advancement of learning. (D. Price, Trans.)* U.K. Cassell & Company.

Bailey, R. N. (1995). Community-oriented primary care programs. *Journal of American Optometric Association, 66*(10), 631–633.

Baker, D. W. (2006). The meaning and measure of health literacy. *Journal of General Internal Medicine, 21*(8), 878–883.

Baker, D. W., Gazmararian, J. A., Williams, M. V., et al. (2002). Functional health literacy and the risk of hospital admission among Medicare managed care enrollees. *American Journal of Public Health, 92*(8), 1278–1283.

Balota, D. A., & Marsh, E. J. (2004). *Cognitive Psychology: Key Readings.* Taylor & Francis. Retrieved from http://lib.myilibrary.com/Browse/open.asp?ID=289 1 5&loc=659.

Bandura, A. (1977). *Social Learning Theory.* New York, NY: General Learning Press.

Bandura, A. (1994). Self-efficacy. In V. S. Ramachaudran (Ed.), *Encyclopedia of human behavior (Vol. 4, pp. 71–81).* New York, NY: Academic Press [Reprinted in H. Friedman [Ed.], Encyclopedia of mental health. San Diego: Academic Press, 1998].

Bandura, A. (1997). *Self-efficacy: The exercise of control.* New York, NY: W.H. Freeman.

Barkhordarian, A., Hacker, B., & Chiappelli, F. (2011). Dissemination of evidence-based standards of care. *Bioinformation, 7*(6), 315–319.

Barlett, E. E. (1986). Historical glimpses of patient education in the United States. *Patient Education and Counseling, 8*(2), 135–149.

Barrett, S. E., & Puryear, J. S. (2006). Health literacy: Improving quality of care in primary care settings. *Journal of Health Care for the Poor and Underserved, 17*(4), 690–697.

Bash, L. (2005). *Best practices in adult learning.* Bolton, MA: Anker Publishing Co.

Bastable, S. B. (2006). *Essentials of Patient Education.* Sudbury, MA: Jones and Barlett.

Bauer, P. J. (1996). What do infants recall of their lives? Memory for specific events by one- to two-year-old. *American Psychologist, 51*(1), 29–41.

Baum, M. (2005). *Understanding behaviorism.* Malden, MA: Blackwell Publishing.

Bayliss, E. A., Ellis, J. L., & Steiner, J. F. (2007). Barriers to self-management and quality-of-life outcomes in seniors with multimorbidities. *Annuals of Family Medicine, 5*(5), 395–402.

Becker, M. H. (Ed.), (1974). The health belief model and personal health behavior. *Health Education Monographs*, *2*(4), 324–473.

Becker, M. H., Kaback, M. M., Rosenstock, I. M., & Ruth, M. V. (1975). Some influences on public participation in a genetic screening program. *Journal of Community Health*, *1*(1), 3–14.

Becker, M. H., Nathanson, C. A., Drachman, R. H., & Kirscht, J. P. (1977). Mothers' health beliefs and children's clinic visits: A prospective study. *Journal of Community Health*, *3*(2), 125–135.

Behar-Horenstein, L. S., Guin, P., Gamble, K., et al. (2005). Improving care through patient and family education programs. *Hospital Topics*, *83*(1), 21–27.

Beisecker, A. E., & Beisecker, T. D. (1990). Patient information-seeking behaviours when communicating with doctors. *Medical Care*, *28*(1), 19–28.

Bell, M. J., Lineker, S. C., Goldsmith, C. H., & Badley, E. M. (1998). A randomized controlled trial to evaluate the efficacy of community based physical therapy in the treatment of people with rheumatoid arthritis. *The Journal of Rheumatology*, *25*(2), 231–237.

Bensing, J. (2000). Bridging the gap: The separate worlds of evidence-based medicine and patient-centered medicine. *Patient Education and Counseling*, *39*(1), 17–25.

Best, J. T. (2001). Effective teaching for elderly: Back to basics. *Orthopaedic Nursing*, *20*(3), 46–52.

Betz, C. L., Ruccione, K., Meeske, K., Smith, K., & Chang, N. (2008). Health literacy: A pediatric nursing concern. *Pediatric Nursing*, *34*(3), 231–239.

Beyer, H. S. (2009). The 300-year-old health care solution. *Archives of Internal Medicine*, *169*(19), 1818.

Billek-Sawhney, B., & Reicherter, E. A. (2005). Literacy and the older adult: Educational considerations for health professionals. *Topics in Geriatric Rehabilitation*, *21*(4), 275–281.

Bishop, G. D. (1991). Understanding the understanding of illness: Lay disease representations. In J. A. Skelton & R. T. Croyle (Eds.), *Mental Representation in Health and Illness* (pp. 32–60). New York: Springer.

Bishop, V. (2009). Leaders of the future. *Nursing Standards*, *24*(10), 62–63.

Bloom, B. (1956). *Taxonomy of educational objectives: The classification of educational goals*. New York, NY: Longman Publishing Group.

Boberg, E. W., Gustafson, D. H., Hawkins, R. P., et al. (2003). Assessing the unmet information, support and care delivery needs of men with prostate cancer. *Patient Education and Counseling*, *49*(3), 233–242.

Bodenheimer, T., & Fernandez, A. (2005). High and rising health care costs: Can costs be controlled while preserving quality? Part 4. *Annals of Internal Medicine*, *143*(1), 26–31.

Bolman, C., Brug, J., Bar, J., & Van de Borne, B. (2005). Long-Term efficacy of a checklist to improve patient education in cardiology. *Patient Education and Counseling*, *56*(2), 240–248.

Boothman, N. (2002). *How to connect in business in 90 seconds or less*. New York, NY: Workman Publishing Company, Inc.

Boreham, P., & Gibson, D. (1978). The informative process in private medical consultations: A preliminary investigation. *Social Science and Medicine*, *12*(5), 409–416.

Boren, S. A., Wakefield, B. J., Gunlock, T. L., & Wakefield, D. S. (2009). Heart failure self-management education: a systematic review of the evidence. *International Journal of Evidence-Based Healthcare*, *7*(3), 159–168.

Boswell, C., Cannon, S., Aung, K., & Eldridge, J. (2004). An application of health literacy research. *Applied Nursing Research*, *17*(1), 61–64.

Bower, G. H., & Hilgard, E. R. (1981). *Theories of learning* (5th ed.). Englewood Cliffs, NJ: Prentice Hall.

Boyd, M. D., Gleit, C. J., Graham, B. A., & Whitman, N. L. (1998). *Health teaching in nursing practice: A professional model* (3rd ed.). Stamford, CT: Appleton & Lange.

Boyde, M., Tuckett, A., Peters, R., Thompson, D., Turner, C., & Stewart, S. (2009). Learning for heart failure patients (The L-HF study). *The Journal of Clinical Nursing*, *18*(14). 2030.

Breslow, L. (1999). From disease prevention to health promote. *Journal of the American Medical Association*, *281*(11), 1030–1033.

Brey, R. A., Clark, S. E., & Wantz, M. S. (2007). Enhancing health literacy through accessing health information, products, and services: An exercise for children and adolescents. *Journal of School Health*, *77*(9), 640–644.

Brey, R. A., Clark, S. E., & Wantz, M. S. (2008). This is your future: A case study approach to foster health literacy. *Journal of School Health*, *78*(6), 351–355.

Brodenheimer, T., Lorig, K., Holman, H., & Grumbach, K. (2002). Patient self-management of chronic disease in primary care. *The Journal of the American Medical Association*, *288*(19), 2469–2475.

Brookfield, S. D. (2006). *The skillful teacher: On technique, trust, and responsiveness in the classroom* (2nd ed.). San Francisco, CA: Jossey-Bass.

Brown, A. L. (1978). Knowing when, where and how to remember: A problem of metacognition. In R. Glaser (Ed.), *Advances in instructional psychology*. Hillsdale, NJ: Erlbaum.

Brown, S. L., Teufel, J. A., & Birch, D. A. (2007). Early adolescents' perceptions of health literacy. *Journal of School Health*, *77*(1), 7–15.

Brunetti, L., & Hermes-DeSantis, E. (2010). The internet as a drug information resource. *US Pharmacist*, *35*, 1. Retrieved December 11, 2011 from http://prod.uspharmacist.corn/content/c/19130/.

Brunner, J. (1990). *Acts of meaning*. Cambridge, MA: Harvard University Press.

Bucy, P. C. (1981). Ancora imparo—I continue to learn. *Neurologia Medico-chirurgica*, *21*(7), 629–634.

Bull, F. C., Kreuter, M. W., & Scharff, D. P. (1999). Effects of tailored, personalized and general health messages on physical activity. *Patient Education and Counseling*, *36*(2), 181–192.

Burnham, E., & Peterson, E. B. (2005). Health information literacy: A library case study. *Library Trends*, *53*(3), 422–433.

Bybee, R. (Ed.), (1966). *National Standards and the Science Curriculum: Challenges, Opportunities, and Recommendations*. Dubuque, Iowa: Kendall-Hunt.

Cagle, J,.G., & Kovacs, P. J. (2009). Education: A complex and empowering social work intervention at end of life. *Health & Social Work*, *34*(1), 17–27.

California State University, Northridge. (2008). *What is a CHES?*. Retrieved from MPH Program http://www.csun.edu/-hchsc006/id42.htm.

Calvin, W. H. (1995). *How brains think: evolving intelligence, then and now.* New York, NY: Basic Books.

Campbell, E. M., Redman, S., Moffitt, P. S., & Sanson-Fisher, R. W. (1996). The relative effectiveness of educational and behavioral instruction programs for patients with NIDDM: A randomized trial. *The Diabetes Educator, 22,* 379–386.

Campbell, R. J. (2008). Meeting seniors' information needs: Using computer technology. *Home Health Care Management and Practice,* (4), 328–335.

Campbell, S. M., Roland, M. O., Middleton, E., & Reeves, D. (2005). Improvements in quality of clinical care in English general practice 1998–2003: Longitudinal observational study. *BMJ, 331,* 1121.

Canadian Public Health Association, Report of Expert panel. (2008). *A vision for a health literate Canada.* Author. Retrieved December 6, 2011, from http://www.cpha.ca/uploads/portals/h-1/report_e.pdf.

Cannick, G. F., Horowitz, A. M., Garr, D. R., et al. (2007). Oral cancer prevention and early detection: Using the PRECEDE-PROCEED framework to guide the training of health professional students. *Journal Of Cancer Education, 22*(4), 250–253.

Carter, N. J., & Wallace, R. L. (2007). Collaborating with public libraries, public health departments, and rural hospitals to provide consumer health information services. *Journal of Consumer Health on the Internet, 11*(4), 1–14.

Center for Health Strategies, Inc. (2005). *What is health literacy? [Fact sheet].* Retrieved from http://www.chcs.org/usr_doc/Health_Literacy_Fact_Sheets.pdf.

Centers for Disease Control. (2007). *Healthy People 2010.* Retrieved from Centers for Disease Control http://www.cdc.gov/nchs/about/otheract/hpdata2010/abouthp.htm.

Chang, B. L., Bakken, S., Brown, S. S., et al. (2004). Bridging the digital divide: Reaching vulnerable populations. *Journal of the American Medical Informatics Association, 11*(6), 448–457.

Chang, M., & Kelly, A. E. (2007). Patient education: Addressing cultural diversity and health literacy issues. *Urologic Nursing, 27*(5), 411–417.

Chase, W. G., & Simon, H. A. (1973). Perception in chess. *Cognitive Psychology, 4,* 55–81.

Chomsky, N. (1959). Review of Skinner's verbal behavior. *Language, 35,* 26–58.

Chulay, M., & Burns, S. M. (2010). *AACN Essentials of Critical Care Nursing* (2nd ed.). New York: McGraw-Hill Professional. Available at: https://search-ebscohost-com.subr.idm.oclc.org/login.aspx?direct=true&db=nlebk&AN=333252&site=eds-live.

Clark, N. M., & Gong, M. (2000). Management of chronic diseases by practitioners and patients: Are we teaching the wrong things? *BMJ, 320,* 572–575.

Clark, N. M., Gong, M., Schork, M. A., et al. (1997). Impact education for physicians on patient outcomes. *Pediatrics, 101*(5), 831–836.

Clark, P. A., Drain, M., & Malone, M. P. (2003). Addressing patients' emotional and spiritual needs. *Joint Commission Journal on Quality and Safety, 29*(12), 659–670.

Close, A. (1988). Patient education: A literature review. *Journal of Advanced Nursing, 13*(2), 203–213.

CMS (2011). *HCACPS: Patients perspectives of care survey.* Retrieved from CMS.gov on December 10, 2011 from https://www.cms.gov/HospitalQualityInits/30_HospitalHCAHPS.asp.

CMS (2016). https://www.cms.gov/medicare/medicare-fee-for-service-payment/.../faq-tcms.pdf.

CMS (2016). *Transitional Care Management Services.* https://www.cms.gov/Outreach-and-Education/Medicare-Learning-Network-MLN/MLNProducts/Downloads/Transitional-Care-Management-Services-Fact-Sheet-ICN908628.pdf.

Coalition of National Health Educators Organizations (CNHEO). (2011). *Profession-wide code of ethics* Available at: http://cnheo.org/ethics-of-the-profession.html.

Coates, H. (2007). *Integrating patient-centered care and evidence-based practices: What is the prognosis for healthcare?.* Indianapolis: (Unpublished research paper) Indiana University. Retrieved December 11, 2011 from http://home.comcast.netl-h.coates/S653-PCC+EBP.pdf.

Cognitivism. (2004). *In Encyclopedia of Applied Psychology.* Retrieved from http://www.credoreference.com/entry/estappliedpsyc/cognitivism.

Collins, A. S., Gullette, D., & Schnepf, M. (2005). Break through language barriers. *Nurse Practitioners: The 2005 sourcebook for advanced practice nurses, 30*(suppl 1), 19–20.

Colombara, F., Martinato, M., Girardin, G., & Gregori, D. (2015). Higher levels of knowledge reduce healthcare costs in patients with inflammatory bowel disease. *Inflammatory Bowel Disease, 21*(3), 615–622.

Committee on Health Literacy. (2004, April 8). *Health Literacy: A prescription to end confusion (The Institute of Medicine of the National Academies).* Washington DC: The National Academies Press.

Committee on Understanding and Eliminating Racial and Ethnic Disparities in Health Care. (2003). *Unequal Treatment: Confronting Racial and Ethnic Disparities in Health Care.* (B.D. Smedley, A. Stith, A. Nelson,) Washington DC: the National Academies Press.

Conti, G., & Welborn, R. (1986). Teaching learning styles and the adult learner. *Lifelong Learning, 9*(8), 20–24.

Cooper, H., Booth, K., Fear, S., & Gill, G. (2001). Chronic disease patient education: Lessons from meta-analyses. *Patient Education and Counseling, 44*(2), 107–117.

Costa, M. L., Rensburg, L. V., & Rushton, N. (2007). Does teaching style matter? A randomised trial of group discussion versus lectures in orthopaedic undergraduate teaching. *Medical Education, 41*(2), 214–217.

Cowan, N. (2001). The magical number of 4 in short-term memory: A reconsideration of mental storage capacity. *Behavioral and Brain Sciences, 24*(1), 87–114.

Cromie, W. J. (2006). *The longer you live the long you can expect to live.* Retrieved from Harvard University Gazette, Retrieved December 11, 2011 http://www.news.harvard.edu/. gazette/2006/07. 20/ 10-deathquiz.html.

Curry, L. C., Walker, C., Hogstel, M. O., & Burns, P. (2005). Teaching older adults to self-manage medications: Preventing adverse drug reactions. *Journal of Gerontological Nursing, 31*(4), 32–42.

Curtis, J. R., Patrick, D. L., Caldwell, E. S., & Collier, A. C. (2000). Why don't patients and physicians talk about end of life care? Barriers to communication for patients with acquired immunodeficiency syndrome and their primary care physician. *Archives of Internal Medicine, 160*(11), 1690–1696.

Cutilli, C. C., & Bennett, I. M. (2009). Understanding the health literacy of America; results of the national assessment of adult literacy. *Orthopaedic Nursing, 28*(1), 27–34.

Czaja, S. J., & Lee, C. C. (2007). The human computer-interaction handbook. In J. A. Jacko & A. Sears (Eds.), *Information Technology and Older Adults* (2nd ed., pp. 777–792). New York: Lawrence Erlbaum.

Davies, K. (2006). What is effective intervention? Using theories of health promotion. *British Journal of Nursing, 15*(5), 252–256.

Davis, P. M. (1991). *Cognition and learning: A review of the literature with reference to ethnolinguistic minorities.* Dallas, TX: Summer Institute of Linguistics.

Davis, T. C., & Wolf, M. S. (2006). Literacy and misunderstanding prescription drug labels. *Annuals of Internal Medicine, 145*(12), 887–894.

Davis, T. C., Berkel, H. J., Arnold, C. L., Nancy, I., Jackson, R. H., & Murphy, P. W. (1998). Intervention study to increase mammography utilization in public health. *Journal of General Internal Medicine, 13*(4), 230–233.

Davis, T. C., Jackson, R. H., George, B. D., et al. (1993). Reading ability in patients in substance misuse treatment centers. *International Journal of the Addictions, 28*(6), 571–582.

DeBrantes, F., Rastogi, A., & Painter, M. (2010). Reducing potentially avoidable approach reducing potentially avoidable complications. *Health Services Research, 45*(6p2), 1854–1871.

Deccache, A., & Aujoulat, I. (2001). A European perspective: Common developments, differences and challenges in patient education. *Patient Education and Counseling, 44*(1), 7–14.

DeGregori, T. R. (2003). Health Issues. *Retrieved from American Council on Science and Health, December, 10,* 2011. http://www.acsh.org/healthissues/newsID.578/healthissue_detail.asp.

Demetriou, A., & Raftopoulos, A. (Eds.), (2005). *Cognitive developmental change: Theories, models and measurement: Cambridge Studies in Cognitive and Perceptual Development.* Cambridge University Press.

Destache, D. M. (2013, April 30). *Hospital policies: Will they be a burden or a benefit to you in litigation? Midwest Legal Advisor.* Dugan and Murray: Lamson.

DeWalt, D. A., Berkman, N. D., Sheridan, S., Lohr, K. N., & Pignone, M. P. (2004). Literacy and health outcomes: A systematic review of the literature. *Journal of General Internal Medicine, 19*(12), 1228–1239.

Dewey, J. (1933). *How we think.: A restatement of the relation of reflective thinking to the educative process.* Chicago, IL: DC Heath Publishing.

Dewey, A., Holecek, A., Sigma Theta Tau International. (2018). *The Nurse's Healthcare Ethics Committee Handbook.* Indianapolis: Sigma.

Deyo, R. A., & Diehl, A. K. (1986). Patient satisfaction with medical care for low back pain. *Spine, 11*(1), 28–30.

Dickens, C., Lambert, B. L., Cromwell, T., & Piano, M. R. (2013). Nurse overestimation of patients' health literacy. *Journal of Health Communication, 18*(Suppl 1), 62–69.

Dictionary, Black's Law, & ed, 6th. (1990). *St. Paul.* Minnesota: West Publishing.

Doak, C. C., Doak, L. G., & Root, J. H. (1995). *Teaching patients with low literacy skills.* Philadelphia, PA: J.B. Lippincott.

Dogra, N., Betancourt, J. R., Park, E. R., & Sprague-Martinez, L. (2009). The relationship between drivers and policy in the implementation of cultural competency training in health care. *Journal of the National Medical Association*, *101*(2), 127–133.

Dube, L., Belanger, M. C., & Trudeau, E. (1996). The role of emotions in health care satisfaction. *Journal of Health Care Marketing*, *16*(2), 45–51.

Durso, F. T., Nickerson, R. S., Dumais, S. T., Lewandowsky, S., & Perfect, T. J. (2007). *Handbook of Applied Cognition*. Wiley. Retrieved from http://lib.myilibrary.com/Browse/open.asp?ID=8387l&Joe=1 78.

Eddy, J. D. (2007). Sequential retrieval and inhibition of parallel (re)activated representations: a neurocomputational comparison of competitive queuing and resampling models. *Adaptive Behavior*, *15*(1), 51–71.

Edmunds, M. (2005). Health literacy: A barrier to patient education. *Nurse Practitioner*, *30*(3), 54.

Ellis, S. E., Speroff, T., Dittus, R. S., Brown, A., Pichert, J. W., & Elasy, T. A. (2004). Diabetes patient education: A met-analysis and meta-regression. *Patient Education and Patient Counseling*, *52*(1), 97–105.

Emanuel, E. J., & Goldman, L. (1998). Protecting patient welfare in managed care: Six safeguards. *Journal of Health Politics, Policy and Law*, *23*(4), 635–639.

Emerson, R. W. (1912). *Journals of Ralph Waldo Emerson: with annotations*. Cambridge, MA: Houghton Mifflin Company.

Engler, A. J. (2005). Maternal stress and the white coat syndrome: A case study. *Pediatric Nursing*, *31*(6), 470–473.

Epstein, R., Franks, P., Fiscella, K., et al. (2005). Measuring patient-centered communication in patient-physician consultations: Theoretical and practical issues. *Social Science and Medicine*, *61*(7), 1516–1528.

Erlen, J. A. (2004). Functional health literacy: Ethical concerns. *Orthopaedic Nursing*, *23*(2), 151–153.

Escalante, C. P., Weiser, M. A., Manzullo, E., et al. (2004). Outcomes of treatment pathways in outpatient treatment of low risk febrile neutropenic cancer patients. *Journal of Supportive Care in Cancer*, *12*(9), 657–662.

Esposito, T. J., Luchette, F. A., & Gamell, R. L. (2006). Do we need neurosurgical coverage in the trauma center? *Advances in Surgery*, *40*, 213–221.

Evans, M. (2004). Poor performance AHA suffers year-end loss for second year in row. *Modern Healthcare*, *34*(38), 9.

Faden, R. R., Becker, C., Lewis, C., Freeman, J., & Faden, A. L. (1981). Disclosure of information to patients in medical care. *Medical Care*, *19*(7), 718–733.

Fallowfield, L., & Jenkins, V. (1999). Effective communication skills are the key to good cancer care. *European Journal of Cancer*, *35*(11), 1592–1597.

Falvo, D. R. (1994). *Effective patient education: A guide to increased compliance* (2nd ed.). Gaithersburg, MD: Aspen.

Falvo, D. R. (2004). *Effective Patient Education: A guide to increased compliance*. Sudbury, MA: Jones and Barlett.

Feldman, J., & McPhee, D. (2008). *The Science of Learning and the Art of Teaching*. Clifton Park, NY: Thomson.

Fishbein, M. (1963). An investigation of relationships between beliefs about an object and the attitude toward that object. *Human Relations*, *16*, 233–240.

Fishbein, M., & Ajzen, I. (1975). *Belief, attitude, intention, and behavior: An intro-duction to theory and research.* Reading, MA: Addison-Wesley.

Fitzgerald, J. T., Funnell, M. M., Hess, G. E., et al. (1998). The reliability and validity of a brief diabetes knowledge test. *Diabetes Care, 21*(5), 706–710.

Fox, S. (2006, October 29). *Pew internet and American life project online health search 2006 [White paper].* Retrieved from Pew Internet http://www.pewinternet. org/PPF/r/190/report_display.asp.

Freeman, S. R., & Chambers, K. A. (1997). Home health care: Clinical pathways and quality integration. *Nursing Management, 28*(6), 45–48.

Friberg, F., Andersson, E. P., & Bengtsson, J. (2007). Pedagogical encounter be-tween nurses and patients in a medical ward-a filed study. *International Journal of Nursing Studies, 44*(4), 534–544.

Friberg, F., Bergh, A. L., & Lepp, M. (2006). In search of details of patient teach-ing in nursing documentation: An analysis of patient records in a medical ward in Sweden. *Journal of Clinical Nursing, 15*(12), 1550–1558.

Funnell, M. M., & Anderson, R. M. (2004). Empowerment and self-management of diabetes. *Clinical Diabetes, 22*(3), 123–127.

Furnee, C. A., Groot, W., & Maassen van den Brink, H. (2008). The health effects of education: A meta-analysis. *Journal of Public Health, 18*(4), 417–421.

Gabbay, M. B., Cowie, V., Kerr, B., & Purdy, B. (2000). Too ill to learn: Double jeopardy in education for sick children. *Journal of Royal Society of Medicine, 93*(3), 114–117.

Galanti, G. (2008). *Caring for Patients from Different Cultures.* Philadelphia, PA: University of Pennsylvania Press.

GAO. (2006). *MEDICARE Communications to Beneficiaries on the Prescription Drug Benefit Could Be Improved.* United States Government Accountability Office.

Gerteis, M., Edgman-Levitan, S., Daley, J., & Delbanco, T. L. (Eds.), (1993). *Through the patient's eyes: understanding and promoting patient-centered care.* New York, NY: Jossey-Bass.

Gessner, B. A. (1989). Adult education: The cornerstone of patient teaching. *The Nursing Clinics of North America, 24*(3), 589–595.

Ginsburg, P. B. (2004). Controlling health care cost. *The New England Journal of Medicine, 351*(16), 1591–1593.

Given, B. K. (2002). *Teaching to the Brain's Natural Learning Systems.* Alexandria, VA.: Association for Supervision and Curriculum Development.

Glanz, K., Rimer, B. K., & Viswanath, K. (2008). *Health behavior and health educa-tion: Theory, research, and practice* (4th ed.). San Francisco, CA: Jossey-Bass.

Glasgow, R. E., Funnell, M. M., Bonomi, A. E., Beckham, V., & Wagner, E. H. (2002). Self-management aspects of the improving chronic care breakthrough series: Implementation with diabetes and heart failure teams. *Annals of Behavioral Medicine, 24*(2), 80–87.

Glasson, J., Chang, E., Chenoweth, L., et al. (2006). Evaluation is a model of nursing care for older patients using participatory action research in an acute medical world. *Journal of Clinical Nursing, 15*(5), 588–598.

Green, L. W., Mercer, S. L., Rosenthal, A. C., Dietz, W. H., & Rusten, C. G. (2003). Possible lessons for physician counselling from the progress in smoking cessation in primary care. In L. Elmadfa, E. Anklam, & J. S. Konig (Eds.), *Modern aspects of nutrition: present knowledge and future perspectives, 56* (pp. 191–194). Basal, Switzerland: Karger Publishers.

Green, C. D. (1994). Cognitivism: Whose party is it anyway? *Canadian Psychology*, *35*(1), 112–123.

Green, L. W., & Kreuter, M. W. (2005). *Health program planning, an educational and ecological approach* (4th ed.). New York, NY: McGraw Hill.

Green, L. W. (2002). Health belief model. In Lester Breslow (Ed.), *Encyclopedia of Public Health* [Vol. 2, pp. 526-528]. New York, NY: Macmillan Reference.

Green, L. W., & Kreuter, M. W. (1991). *Health Promotion Planning: An Educational and Environmental Approach* (2nd ed.). Palo Alto, CA: Mayfield Publishing.

Greenburg, D. (2001). A critical look at health literacy. *Adult Basic Education*, *11*(2), 67–79.

Greenburg, L. A. (1991). Teaching children who are learning disabled about illness and hospitalization. *The American Journal of Maternal/Child Nursing*, *16*(5), 260–263.

Greene, M. G., & Adelman, R. D. (2003). Physician-older patient communication about cancer. *Patient Education and Counseling*, *50*(1), 55–60.

Griggs, T. (2011). Communication Key to Patient Education. In *Louisiana Medical News*. Retrieved from: http://www.louisianamedicalnews.com/mod/secfile/viewed.php?file_id=65.

Gross domestic report: Third quarter 2009. (2009, December 22). *U.S. Department of Commerce*. Retrieved January 18, 2010, from Bureau of Economic Analysis National Economic Accounts http://www.bea.gov/newsreleases/national/gdp/2009/pdf/gdp3q09 3rd.pdf.

Guadagnoli, E., & Ward, P. (1998). Patient-participation in decision-making. *Social Sciences and Medicine*, *47*(3), 329–339.

Guevara, J. P., Wolf, F., Grum, C. M., & Clark, N. M. (2003). Effect of educational interventions for self-management of asthma in children and adolescents: systematic review and meta-analysis. *British Medical Journal*, *326*(7402), 1308–1309.

Gura, M. T. (2004). *Clinical considerations for the allied professional: Standards of professional practice for the allied professional in electrophysiology and pacing*. *Heart Rhythm*, *1*(4), 250–251.

Gustafson, D. H., Arora, N. K., Nelson, E. C., & Boberg, E. W. (2003). Increasing understanding of patient needs during and after hospitalization. *Joint Commission Journal on Quality and Safety*, *27*(2), 81–92.

Hahn, S. R. (2009). Patient-centered communication to assess and enhance patient adherence to glaucoma medication. *Ophthalmology*, *116*(11), S37–S42.

Hall, J. A., Roter, D. L., & Katz, N. R. (1988). Meta-analysis of correlates of provider behavior in medical encounters. *Medical Care*, *26*(7), 657–675.

Hamilton, N. (2005). Grief and bereavement: Coping with loss of a spouse. *Nursing and Residential Care*, *7*(5), 214–216.

Hanchate, A. D., Ashe, A. S., Gazmarian, J. A., Wolf, M. S., & Paasche-Orlow, M. K. (2008). The demographic assessment for health literacy (DAHL): A new tool for estimating associations between health literacy and outcomes in national surveys. *Journal of General Internal Medicine*, *23*(10), 1561–1566.

Hanks, G. (1994). The effect of healthcare reform on academic medicals. *The International Journal of Radiation Oncology Biology Physics*, *31*(4), 999–1004.

Harlan, L. (2007). Under pressure. *Network Journal*, *14*(7), 36. Retrieved from Ethnic NewsWatch (ENW). http://dx.doi.org/ 1367503711.

Harper, W. (2007). Teaching health literacy: Building a foundation for safer health care. *Focus on Patient Safety Newsletter, 10*(1), 5–6.

Harper, W., Cook, S., & Makoul, G. (2007). Teaching students about health literacy: 2 Chicago initiatives. *American Journal of Healthy Behavior, 31*(Suppl. 1), S111–S114.

Canada, Health. (1999). *Toward a healthy future: Second report on the health of Canadians [White paper].* Retrieved from Public Health Agency of Canada. http://www.hc-sc.gc.ca/hppb/phdd/report/text_versions/english/index.html.

Canada, Health. (1999). *Toward a healthy future: Second report on the health of Canadians.* Retrieved from http://www.hc-sc.gc.ca/hppb/phdd/report/text_versions/english/index.html.

Heisler, M., Bouknight, R. R., Hayward, R. A., & Smith, D. M. (2002). The relative importance of physician communication, participatory decision making, and patient understanding in diabetes self-management. *Journal of General Internal Medicine, 17*(4), 249–252.

Henderson, S. (2002). Influences on patient participation and decision-making in care. *Professional Nurse, 17*(9), 521–525.

Hernandez, P., Balter, M., Bourbeau, J., & Hodder, R. (2009). Living with chronic obstructive pulmonary disease: A survey of patients' knowledge and attitudes. *Respiratory Medicine, 103*(1), 1004–1012.

Hess, T. M., & Tate, C. S. (1991). Adult age differences in explanations and memory for behavioral information. *Psychology and Aging, 6*(1), 86–92.

Hesse, B. W., Nelson, D. E., Kreps, G. L., et al. (2005). Trust and sources of health information: The impact of the Internet and its implications for health care providers: Findings from the first Health Information National Trends Survey. *Archives of Internal Medicine, 165*(22), 2618–2624.

Hiemstra, R., & Sisco, B. (1990). *Individualizing Instruction.* San Francisco, CA: Jossey-Bass.

Higbee, H. L. (2001). *Your memory: how it works and how to improve it.* New York: Da Capo Press.

Hilgard, E. R. (1988). Review of BF Skinner's the behavior of organisms. *Journal of the Experimental Analysis of Behavior, 50*(2), 283–286.

Hill, A., McPhail, S., Hoffmann, T., et al. (2009). A randomized trial comparing digital video disc with written delivery of falls prevention education for older patients in hospitals. *Journal of Geriatric Society, 57*(8), 1458–1463.

Hill, E. K. (2005). Assessing health literacy: Providing useable health information for seniors at discharge in northern Idaho. *Journal of Hospital Librarianship, 5*(4), 11–24.

Hill, R., & Dunbar, R. (2002). Social network size in humans. *Human Nature, 14*(1), 53–72.

Hirsch, E. D. (1988). *Cultural literacy: What every American needs to know.* New York: Vintage Books.

Hoare, C. (2006). *Handbook of adult development and learning.* New York, NY: Oxford University Press.Jensen, E. (2000). *Brain-based learning.* Thousand Oaks, CA; Corwin Press.

Hoffman, T., & McKenna, K. (2006). Analysis of stroke patients' and carers' reading ability and the content and design of written materials: Recommendations for improving written stroke information. *Patient Education and Counseling, 60*(3), 286–293.

Houts, P. S., Bachrach, R., Witmer, J. T., Tringali, C. A., Bucher, J. A., & Localio, R. A. (1998). Using pictographs to enhance recall of medical instructions. *Patient Education and Counseling, 35*(2), 83–88.

Houts, P. S., Witmer, J. T., Egeth, H. E., Loscalzo, M. J., & Zabora, J. R. (2000). Using pictographs to enhance recall of medical instructions II. *Patient Education and Counseling, 43*(3), 231–232.

Hoving, C., Visser, A., Mullen, P. D., & van den Borne, B. (2010). A history of patient education by health professionals in Europe and North America: From authority to shared decision making education. *Patient Education and Counseling, 78*(3), 275–281.

Howard, D. H., Gazmararian, J., & Parker, R. M. (2005). The impact of low health literacy on the medical costs of Medicare managed care enrollees. *The American Journal of Medicine, 118*(4), 371–377.

Howard, D. H., Sentell, T., & Gazmararian, J. A. (2006). Impact of health literacy on socioeconomic and racial differences in health in an elderly population. *Journal of General Internal Medicine, 21*(8), 857–861.

Hutchinson, T. A., Hutchinson, N., & Arnaert, A. (2009). Whole person care: Encompassing the two faces of medicine. *Canadian Medical Association Journal, 180*(8), 845–846.

Hwang, S. W., Tram, C. Q., & Knarr, N. (2005). The effect of illustrations on patient comprehension of medication instruction labels. *BMC Family Practice, 16*(6), 26–32.

Iacono, J., & Campbell, A. (1997). *Patient and Family Education: The Compliance Guide to JCAHO Standards.* Marblehead, MA: HCpro.

Institute of Medicine Committee on the Health Professions Education Summit (2003). Greiner AC, Knebel E, editors. *Health Professions Education: A Bridge to Quality.* Washington, DC: National Academies Press. Available at: https://www.ncbi.nlm.nih.gov/books/NBK221528.

Institute of Medicine of the National Academies. (2009). *Toward Health Equity and Patient-Centeredness: Integrating Health Literacy, Disparities Reduction, and Quality Improvement.* Washington, D.C.: The National Academies Press.

Institute of Medicine. (2002). Committee on Communication for Behavior Change in the 21st Century. In *Speaking of Health: Assessing Health Communication Strategies for Diverse Populations.* Washington, DC: National Academies Press.

Jenkins, V., & Fallowfield, L. (2002). Can communication skills training alter physicians' beliefs and behavior in clinic? *Journal of Clinical Oncology, 20*(3), 765–769.

Jenkins, V., Fallowfield, L., & Saul, J. (2001). Information needs of patients with cancer: Results from a large study in UK cancer centers. *British Journal of Cancer, 84*(1), 48–51.

Jensen, E. (2000). *Brain-based learning: the new science of teaching and learning.* Thousand Oaks, CA: Corwin Press.

Jervey, G. M. (2001). *American Medical Association Journal of Ethics.* Retrieved from Virtual Mentor http://virtualmentor.ama-assn.org/2001/04/prsp 1-0104.html.

Johannessen, B. (2010). *One Answer to Louisiana's Poor Health Rankings.* Retrieved on December 12, 2011 from http://www.lhcrmedicare.org/CareTransitionsInnovationAward.html.

Jones, F. (2000). *Tools for teaching.* Santa Cruz, CA: Fredric Jones & Associates.

Jones, S., & Fox, S. (2009). *Pew Research Center*. Retrieved from Pew Internet http://pewinternet.org/Reports/2009/Generations-Online-in-2009.aspx.

Karpf, M., Lofgren, R., & Perman, J. (2009). Health care reform and its potential impact on academic medical centers. *Academic Medicine, 84*(11), 1472–1475.

Kasmael, P., Atrkar-Roushan, Z., Majlesi, F., & Joker, F. (2008). Mother's knowledge about acute rheumatic fever. *Paediatric Nursing, 20*(9), 32–34.

Kaufman, J. (2008). Patients as partners. *Nursing Management, 39*(8), 45.

Kaye, M. (2009). *Health literacy and informatics in the geriatric population: The challenges and opportunities*. Retrieved from Online Journal of Nursing Informatics http://ojni.org/13_3/Kaye.pdf.

Kelly, P., & Haidet, P. (2007). Physician overestimation of patient literacy: A potential source of health care disparities. *Patient Education and Counseling, 66*(1). 199–122.

Kerr, M. (2008). Do I have white coat syndrome? *Irish Times, 16*. http://dx.doi.org/ 1514464341.

Kessels, R. P. (2003). Patients' memory for medical information. *Journal of the Royal Society of Medicine, 96*(5), 219–222.

Keulers, B. J., Schelting, M. R., Houterman, S., Van Der Wilt, G. J., & Spauwen, P. H. (2008). Surgeons underestimate their patients' desire for preoperative information. *World Journal of Surgery, 32*(6), 964–970.

Kick, E. (1989). Patient teaching for elders. *The Nursing Clinics of North America, 24*(3), 681–686.

Kiekbusch, I. S. (2001). Health literacy: Addressing the health and education divide. *Health Promotion International, 16*(3), 289–297.

Kindelan, K., & Kent, G. (1987). Concordance between patients' information preferences and general practitioners' perceptions. *Psychology and Health, 1*(4), 399–409.

Kinnersley, P., Edwards, A., Hood, K., et al. (2008). Interventions before consultations to help patients address their information needs by encouraging question asking: Systematic review. *British Medical Journal, 337*(7662), 335–339.

Kirsch, S., Jungeblut, A., Jenkins, L., & Kolstad, A. (2002, April). *Adult literacy in America: A first look at the findings of the National Adult Literacy Survey (NCES 1993-275)*. Retrieved from National Center for Educational Statistics http://nces.ed.gov/pubs93/93275.pdf.

Kirscht, J. P., Haefner, D. P., Kegeles, S. S., & Rosenstock, I. M. (1966). A national study of health beliefs. *Journal of Health and Human Behavior, 7*(4), 243–254.

Klein, S. B. (2009). *Learning Principles and Applications* (5 ed.). Thousand Oaks, CA: Sage.

Knowles, M. S. (1950). *Informal Adult Education: A Guide for Administrators, Leaders, and Teachers*. New York, NY: Association Press.

Knowles, M. S. (1968). Andragogy, not pedagogy. *Adult Leadership, 16*(10), 350–352. 386.

Knowles, M. S. (1973). *The adult learner: A neglected species*. Houston: Gulf Publishing.

Knowles, M. S. (1975). *Self-directed learning: A guide for learners and teachers*. Englewood Cliffs, NJ: Prentice Hall/Cambridge.

Knowles, M. S. (1977). *The adult education movement in the United States*. Malabar, FL: Krieger.

Knowles, M. S. (1980). *The modern practice of adult education: From pedagogy to andragogy*. Englewood Cliffs, NJ: Prentice Hall/Cambridge.

Knowles, M. S. (1984). *Andragogy in action: Applying modern principles of adult education*. San Francisco, CA: Jossey-Bass.

Knowles, M. S. (1984). *The adult learner: A neglected species* (3rd ed.). Houston, TX: Gulf.

Knowles, M. S. (1990). *The adult learner: A neglected species* (4th ed.). Houston, TX: Gulf.

Knowles, M. S., Holton, E. F., & Swanson, R. A. (2005). *The adult learner: the definitive classic in adult education and human resource development* (6th ed.). San Diego, CA: Elsevier.

Korsch, B. M., Gozzi, E. K., & Francis, V. (1968). Gaps in doctor-patient communication. *Pediatrics, 42*(5), 855–871.

Krathwohl, D. R., Bloom, B. S., & Masia, B. B. (1964). *Taxonomy of educational objectives book 2: Affective domain*. New York, NY: David McKay.

Kraut, J. (Ed.), (1981). *American Jurisprudence (2nd ed., Vol. 61)*. Rochester, NY: The Lawyer's Cooperative.

Kravitz, R. L., Bell, R. A., Azari, R., Krupat, E., Kelly-Reif, S., & Thom, D. (2002). Request fulfillment in office practice: Antecedents and relationship to outcomes. *Medical Care, 40*(1), 38–51.

Kripalani, S., & Weiss, B. D. (2006). Teaching about health literacy and clear communication. *Journal of General Internal Medicine, 21*(8), 888–890.

Kripalani, S., Henderson, L. E., Chiu, E. Y., Robertson, R., Kolm, P., & Jacobson, T. (2006). Predictors of medication self-management skill in a low literacy population. *Journal of General Internal Medicine, 21*(8), 852–856.

Kübler-Ross, E. (1969). *On death and dying*. New York, NY: Macmillan.

Kubler-Ross, E., & Kessler, D. (2005). *On grief and grieving: finding the meaning of grief through the five stages of loss*. New York, NY: Simon and Schuster.

Kurashige, E. M. (2008). Health literacy: What are the organizational barriers and concerns? *AAACN Viewpoint*, 3–4.

Kutner, M. A. (2006). The health history of America's adults: [electronic resource]: results from the 2003 National Assessment of Adult Literacy. U.S. Department of Education, National Center for Education Statistics. Retrieved from https://nces. ed.gov/pubsearch/pubsinfo.asp?pubid=2006483.

Lahaie, U. (2008). Is nursing ready for webquests? *Journal of Nursing Education, 47*(12), 567–570.

Lainscak, M., & Keber, I. (2005). Validation of self-assessment patient knowledge questionnaire for heart failure patients. *European Journal pf Cardiovascular Nursing, 4*(4), 269–272.

Lambrew, J. M. (2004). Numbers matter: A guide to cost and coverage estimates in health reform debates. *The Journal of Law, Medicine, and Ethics, 32*(3), 446–453.

Lancaster, G. I., O'Connell, R., Katz, D. L., et al. (2009). The expanding medical and behavioral resources with access to care for everyone health plan. *Annals of Internal Medicine, 150*(7), 490–492.

Leanne, A., Andrea, M., & Wendy, C. (2008). Health literacy in the United States. *Critical Care Nurse, 28*(4), 10.

Lefrancois, G. (1995). *Theories of human learning: Kro's report* (3rd ed.). Pacific Grove, CA: Brooks/Cole.

Lenhart, A., Simon, M., & Graziano, M. (2001). *The Internet and Education: Findings of the Pew Internet and American Life Project.* Washington, D.C.: Pew Internet and American Life Project.

Leonard, K. J., & Wilijer, D. (2007). Patient are destined to manage their care. *Healthcare Quarterly, 10*(3), 76–78.

Levinson, W., Gorawara-Bhat, R., & Lamb, J. (2000). A study of patient clues and physician responses in primary care and surgical settings. *Journal of the American Medical Association, 284*(8), 1021–1027.

Levinson, W., Gorawara-Bhat, R., Daeck, R., et al. (1999). Resolving disagreements in the patient-physician relationship: Tools for improving communication in managed care. *Journal of the American Medical Association, 282*(15), 1477–1483.

Levy-Storms, L. (2008). Therapeutic communication training in long term care interventions: Recommendations for future research. *Patient Education and Counseling, 73*(1), 8–21.

Lewis, M., Gohagan, I., & Merenstein, D. The locality rule and the physician's dilemma. Available at: https://www.rwjf.org/en/library/research/2007/06/the-locality-rule-and-the-physician-s-dilemma.html.

Leydon, G. M., Boulton, M., Moynihan, C., et al. (2000). Cancer patients' information needs and information seeking behaviour: In depth study. *British Medical Journal, 320*(7239), 909–913.

Lidell, E., & Fridlund, B. (1996). Long-term effects of comprehensive rehabilitation programme after myocardial infarction. *Scandinavian Journal of Caring Sciences, 10*(2), 67–74.

Lineker, S. C., Bell, M. J., Wilkins, A. L., & Bradley, E. M. (2001). Improving the following short-term home-based physical therapy are maintained at one year for people with moderate to severe rheumatoid arthritis. *Journal of Rheumatology, 28*, 165–168.

Lineker, S. C., Bradley, E. M., Hughes, E. A., & Bell, M. J. (1997). Development of an instrument to measure knowledge in individuals with rheumatoid arthritis: The ACREAU rheumatoid arthritis knowledge inventory questionnaire. *Journal of Rheumatology, 24*(4), 647–653.

Lofgen, R., Karpf, M., Perman, J., & Higdon, C. M. (2006). The US health care systems is in crisis: Implications for academic medical centers and their missions. *Academic Medicine, 81*(8), 713–720.

London, F. (n.d.). *No time to teach? A nurse's guide to patient and family education.* Philadelphia, PA: Lippincott Williams and Wilkins.

Longtin, Y., Say, H., Leape, L. L., Sheridan, S. E., Donaldson, L., & Pittet, D. (2010). Patient participation: Current knowledge and application to patient safety. *Mayo Clinic Proceedings, 1*, 53–62.

Lord, T. R. (1997). A comparison between traditional and constructivist teaching in college biology. *Innovative Higher Education, 21*(3), 197–216.

Lorenzen, B., Melby, C. E., & Earles, B. (2008). Using principles of health literacy to enhance informed consent process. *Association of Operating Room Nursing Journal, 88*(1), 23–29.

Lorig, K. (1992). *Patient education: a practical approach. St.* Louis, MO: Mosby Year Book.

Luker, K., & Caress, A. L. (1989). Rethinking patient education. *Journal of Advance Nursing, 14*(9), 711–718.

Lund, C. H., Carruth, A. K., Moody, K. B., & Logan, C. A. (2005). Theoretical approaches to motivating change: A farm family case example. *American Journal of Health Education, 36*(5), 279–285.

MacGregor, J. N. (1987). Short-term memory capacity: Limitation or optimization. *Psychological Review, 94*(1), 107–108.

Maeland, J., & Havik, O. (1987). Psychological predictors for return to work after a myocardial infarction. *Journal of Psychosomatic Research, 31,* 471–481.

Maeland, J. G., & Havik, O. E. (1987). Measuring cardiac health knowledge. *Scandinavian Journal of Caring Sciences, 1*(1), 23–31.

Maeland, J. G., & Havik, O. E. (1987). The effects of an in-hospital educational programme for myocardial infarction patients. *Scandinavian Journal of Rehabilitation Medicine, 19*(2), 57–65.

Maguire, P., Booth, K., Elliot, C., & Jones, B. (1996). Helping health professionals involved in cancer care acquire key interviewing skills- the impact of workshops. *European Journal of Cancer, 32*(9), 1486–1488.

Maguire, P., Fairbarin, S., & Fletcher, C. (1986). Consultation skills of young doctors: Benefits of feedback training in interviewing as students persist. *British Medical Journal, 292*(14), 1573–1576.

Maibach, E. W., Van Duyn, M. S., & Bloodgood, B. (2006). *A marketing perspective on disseminating evidence-based approaches to disease prevention and health promotion.* Retrieved December 8, 2011, from CDC http://www.cdc.gov/pcd/issues/2006/jul/05_0154.htm.

Major, G., & Homes, J. (2007). How do nurses describe health care procedures? Analysing nurse-patient interaction in a hospital ward. *Australian Journal of Advanced Nursing, 25*(4), 58–70.

Makelainen, P., Vehvilainen-Julkunen, K., & Pietila, A. M. (2008). A survey of rheumatoid arthritis patients' self-efficacy. *Internet Journal of Advanced Nursing Practice, 9*(2), 6.

Makoul, G. (2003). The interplay between education and research about patient-provider communication. *Patient Education and Counseling, 50,* 79–84.

Makoul, G., Arnston, P., & Schofield, T. (1995). Health promotion in primary care: Physician-patient communication and decision making about prescription medications. *Social Science and Medicine, 41*(9), 1241–1254.

Mancuso, J. M. (2008). Health literacy: A concept/dimensional analysis. *Nursing and Health Sciences, 10,* 248–255.

Maniaci, M. J., Heckman, M. G., & Dawson, N. L. (2008). Functional health literacy and understanding of medications at discharge. *Mayo Clinic Proceedings, 83*(5), 554–558.

Manning, K. D., & Kripalani, S. (2007). The use of standardized patients to teach low literacy communication. *American Journal of Healthy Behavior, 31*(Suppl. 1), Sl05–S110.

Marcus, E. N. (2006). The Silent Epidemic-The Health Effects of Illiteracy. *New England Journal of Medicine, 355*(4), 339–341.

Marcus, C. (2014). Strategies for improving the quality of verbal patient and family education: a review of the literature and creation of the EDUCATE model. *Health Psychology and Behavioral Medicine, 2*(1), 482–495.

Markus, K. (1997). *Issues in Ethics home page. Retrieved from Santa Clara University December 2011.* http://www.scu.edu/ethics/publications/iie/v8nl/advancedirectives.html.

Marr, D. (1971). Simple memory: A theory for archicortex. *Philosophical Transactions of the Royal Society of London B, 262*(84), 23–81.

Mayer, G. G., & Villaire, M. (2007). *Health literacy in primary care: A clinician's guide.* New York, NY: Springer.

Mayer, R. E. (1987). *Educational psychology: A cognitive approach.* Boston, MA: Little Brown.

Mcintosh, W., & Kubena, K. (1996). An application of the health belief model to reductions in fat and cholesterol intake. *Journal of Wellness Perspectives, 12*(2), 98.

McKenzie, J. (2000). Information needs of patients with cancer: Similar study had similar findings. *British Medical Journal, 321*(7261), 632.

McLaughlin, N. (2008). The 2008 greeders' cup: Distress in financial markets can be blamed on fiscal irresponsibility. *Modern Healthcare, 38*(38), 41.

McPhee, J. T., Asham, E. H., Rohrer, M. J., et al. (2007). The midterm results of stent graft treatment of thoracic aortic injuries. *Journal of Surgical Research, 138*(2), 181–188.

Meek, R., Kelly, A., & Hu, X. (2009). Use of the visual analog scale to rate and monitor severity of nausea in the emergency department. *Academic Emergency Medicine, 16*(12), 1304–1310.

Merriam, S. B., & Caffarella, R. S. (1991). *Learning in adulthood: A comprehensive guide.* New York, NY: Jossey Bass.

Mikulic, M. (2019). U.S. Health Expenditure as Percent of GDP 1960–2019.

Miller, G. A. (1956). The magical number seven, plus or minus two: Some limits on our capacity for processing information. *Psychological Review, 63*(2), 81–97.

Miller, N. H., Hill, M., Kottke, T., & Ockene, L. S. (1997). The multilevel compliance challenge: Recommendations for a call to action. *Circulation, 95,* 1085–1090.

Miller, W. R., & Rollnick, S. (2002). *Motivational Interviewing: Preparing People to Change.* New York, NY: Guilford Press.

Minninger, J. (1997). *Total recall: How to maximize your memory power.* New York, NY: MJF Books.

Mitchell, G., Murray, J., & Hynson, J. (2008). Understanding the whole person: Life limiting illness across the life span. In G. Mitchell (Ed.), *Palliative Care: A Patient-Centered Approach* (pp. 79–107). Oxon, U.K.: Radcliffe Publishing, Ltd.

Monachos, C. L. (2007). Assessing and addressing low health literacy among surgical outpatients. *AORN Journal, 86*(3), 373–383.

Mondale, S., & Patton, S. B. (2001). *The Story of American Public Education.* Boston, MA: Beacon Press.

Moons, P., DeVolder, E., Budts, W., DeGeest, S., Elen, J., Waeytens, K., et al., (2001). What do patients with congenital heart disease know about their disease, treatment and prevention of complications?: A call for structured patient education. *Heart, 86*(1), 74–80.

Mordiffi, S. Z., Tan, S. P., & Wong, M. K. (2003). Information provided to surgical patients verses information needed. *AORN Journal, 77*(3), 546–562.

Morrow, D. G., Weiner, M., Young, J., Steinley, D., Deer, M., & Murray, M. D. (2005). Improving medication knowledge among older adults with heart failure: A patient centered approach to instruction design. *The Gerontologist, 45*(4), 545–552.

Mullen, P. D., Simons-Morton, D. G., Ramfrez, G., Frankowski, F., Green, L. W., & Mains, D. A. (1997). A meta-analysis of trails evaluating patient education and counseling for three groups of preventive health behaviors. *Patient Education and Counseling, 32*(3), 157–173.

Murray, M. D., & Callahan, C. M. (2003). Improving medication use for older adults: An integrated research agenda. *Annuals of Internal Medicine, 139*(5), 425–429.

Myers, J., & Pellino, T. (2009). Developing new ways to address learning needs of adult abdominal organ transplant recipients. *Progress In Transplantation, 19*(2), 160–166.

Nasaw, D. (1979). *Schooled to Order: A social history of public schooling in the United States.* Oxford, U.K.: Oxford University Press.

National Health Expenditure Data. (2010). Retrieved from Centers for Medicare and Medicaid Services http://www.cms.hhs.gov/NationalHealthExpendData/25_NHE_Fact_Sheet.asp.

National League of Nursing (NLN). (1976). *Patient Education.* New York, NY: NLN.

National Patient Safety Foundation (n.d.). *Ask Me 3 Program.* Retrieved from http://www.npsf.org/askme3/for_patients.php.

Forum, National Quality. (2005). *Implementing a national voluntary consensus standard for informed consent [Brochure].* Washington, D.C.: Author.

Noddings, N. (2006). Educational leaders as caring teachers. *School Leadership & Management, 26*(4), 339–345.

Novak, J. (1998). *Learning, creating and using knowledge: Concept maps as teaching tools in schools and corporations.* Mahwah, NJ: Lawrence Erlbaum Associates.

Nutbeam, D. (2000). Health literacy as a public health goal: A challenge for contemporary health education and communication strategies into the 21st century. *Health Promotion International, 15*(3), 259–267.

O'Keefe, J. H., Carter, M. D., & Lavie, C. J. (2009). Primary and secondary prevention of cardiovascular diseases: a practical evidence-based approach. *Mayo Clinic Proceedings, 84*(8), 741–757.

Oliver, J. W., Kravtiz, R. L., Kaplan, S. H., & Meyers, F. J. (2001). Individualized patient education and coaching to improve pain control among cancer outpatients. *Journal of Clinical Oncology, 19*(8), 2206–2212.

Ong, L. M., Visser, M. R., Lammes, F. B., & de Raes, J. C. (2000). Doctor-patient communication and cancer patients' quality of life and satisfaction. *Patient Education and Counseling, 41*(2), 145–156.

Ormrod, J. E. (1999). *Human learning.* Upper Saddle River, NJ: Prentice Hall.

Ormrod, J. E. (2008). *Human learning* (5th ed.). Columbus, OH: Prentice Hall.

Osborn, C. Y., Weiss, B. D., Davis, T. C., Skripkauskas, S., Rodrique, C., Bass, P. F., et al. (2007). Measuring adult literacy in health care: Performance of the newest vital sign. *American Journal of Health Behavior, 31*(1), 37–45.

Osborne, H. (2005). *Health literacy from A to Z: Practical ways to communicate your health message.* Sudbury, MA: Jones and Barlett.

Overskeid, G. (1995). Cognitivist or behaviorist-who can tell the difference? The case of implicit and explicit knowledge. *British Journal of Psychology, 86*(4), 517.

Paasche-Orlow, M. K., Parker, R. M., Gazmarain, J. A., Nielsen-Bohlan, L. T., & Rudd, R. R. (2005). The prevalence of limited health literacy. *Journal of General Internal Medicine, 20*(2), 175–184.

Paasche-Orlow, M. K., Schillinger, D., Greene, S. M., & Wagner, E. H. (2006). How health care systems can begin to address the challenge of limited literacy. *Journal of General Internal Medicine, 21*(8), 884–887.

Palazzo, M. O. (2009). Patient and Family Education in Critical Care. In P. Morton & D. Fontaine (Eds.), *Critical care nursing: a holistic approach.* New York, NY: Lippincott Williams & Wilkins.

Parikh, N. S., Parker, R. M., Nurss, J. R., Baker, D. W., & Williams, M. V. (1996). Shame and health literacy: The unspoken connection. *Patient Education and Counseling, 27*(1), 33–39.

Parker, R. M., Ratzan, S. C., & Lurie, N. (2003). Health literacy: A policy challenge for advance high-quality health care. *Health Affairs, 22*(4), 147–153.

Pavlov, I. P. (1927). *Conditioned reflexes: An investigation of the physiological activity of the cerebral cortex.* Retrieved from *Classics in the History of Psychology* http://psychclassics.yorku.ca/Pavlov/.

Pawlak, R. (2005). Economic considerations of health literacy. *Nursing Economics, 23*(4), 173–180.

Pender, N.J., Murdaugh, C.L., & Parsons, M.A. (2002). *Assumptions and theoretical propositions of the health promotion model.* Retrieved from University of Michigan Web Site: http://www.nursing. umich,edu/faculty/pender/HPM.pdf.

Penzo, J. A., & Harvey, P. (2008). Understanding parental grief as a response to mental illness: Implications for practice. *Journal of Family Social Work, 11*(3), 323–338.

Perry, L. (2006). Promoting evidence-based practice in stroke care in Australia. *Nursing Standard, 20*(34), 35–42.

Peterson, S. J., & Bredow, T. S. (2009). *Middle range theories: Application to nursing research* (2nd ed.). Philadelphia, PA: Lippincott Williams & Wilkins.

Phillips, L. D. (1999). Patient education: Understanding the process to maximize time and outcomes. *Journal of Intravenous Nursing, 22*(1), 19–35.

Piaget, J. (1954). *The construction of reality in the child.* New York, NY: Basic Books.

Piaget, J. (1967). *Biology and Knowledge.* Chicago, IL: University of Chicago Press.

Piaget, J. (1977). *The Essential Piaget.* New York, NY: Basic Books.

Piaget, J. (1983). Piaget's theory. In P. Mussen (Ed.), *Handbook of Child Psychology,* 4(1). New York, NY: Wiley.

Piaget, J. (1995). *Sociological Studies.* London, U.K.: Routledge.

Pickert, K. (2010). *The unsustainable U.S. health care system, time: Swampland.* Retrieved December 8, 2011 from http://swampland.time.com/2010/02/04/theunsustainable-u-s-health-care-system/.

Pierce, P. F., & Hicks, F. D. (2001). Patient decisions making behavior: An emerging paradigm for nursing science. *Nursing Research, 50*(5), 267–274.

Piette, J. D., Heisler, M., & Wagner, T. H. (2004). Cost-related medication underuse. *Archives of Internal Medicine, 164*(16), 1749–1755.

Pignone, M., DeWalt, D. A., Sheridan, S., Berkman, N., & Lohr, K. N. (2005). Interventions to improve health outcomes for patients with low literacy: A systematic review. *Journal of General Internal Medicine, 20*(2), 185–192.

Piotrowski, N. A. (2005). *Psychology Basics.* Salem Press. Retrieved from http://lib. myilibrary.com/Browse/open.asp?ID=9704l&loc=498.

Polit, D. F., & Beck, C. T. (2006). *Essentials of nursing research: Methods, appraisal, and utilization* (6th ed.). Philadelphia, PA: Lippincott Williams and Wilkins.

Prasauskas, R., & Spoo, L. (2006). Literally Improving Patient Health Outcomes. *Home Health Care Management Practice, 18*(4), 270–327.

Price, D. (1893). *The advancement of learning by Francis Bacon.* U.K.: Cassell & Company.

Prilleltensky, I. (2005). Promoting well-being: Time for a paradigm shift in health and human services. *Scandinavian Journal of Public Health, 66,* 53–60.

Pring, R. (2004). The skills revolution. *Oxford Review Of Education, 30*(1), 105–116.

Prochaska, J. O. (2009). Flaws in theory or flaws in the study. *A commentary on the effect of transtheoretical model based inventions on smoking cessation, 68*(3), 407–409.

Prochaska, J. O., & Velicer, W. F. (1997). The transtheoretical model of health behavior change. *American Journal of Health Promotion, 12*(1), 38–48.

Prossier, H., Almond, S., & Walley, T. (2003). Influences on GPs' decision to prescribe new drugs: The importance of who says what. *Family Practice, 20*(1), 61–68.

Quirk, M., Mazor, K., Haley, H., Philbin, M., Fischer, M., Sullivan, K., et al. (2008). How patients perceive a doctor's caring attitude. *Patient education and counseling, 72*(3), 359–366.

Raczynski, J. M., & DiClemente, R. J. (1999). *Handbook of Health Promotion and Disease Prevention.* New York: Kluwer Academic/Plenum.

Ramey, C. (2005). Did God create psychologists in His image? Re-conceptualizing cognitivism and the subject matter of psychology. *Journal of Theoretical and Philosophical Psychology, 25*(2), 173–190.

Rankin, S. H., & Stallings, K. D. (1996). *Patient education: Issues, principles, practices* (3rd ed.). Philadelphia, PA: Lippincott.

Rankin, S. H., & Stallings, K. D. (2001). *Patient Education: Issues, principles, practices* (4th ed.). Philadelphia, PA: Lippincott-Raven.

Rankin, S. H., Stallings, K. D., & London, F. (2005). *Patient Education in Health and Illness* (5th ed.). Philadelphia, PA: Lippincott Williams and Wilkins.

Raynor, D. K. (2008). Medication literacy in a 2-way street. *Mayo Clinic Proceedings, 83*(5), 520–522.

Redman, B. K. (2001). *The practice of patient education* (9th ed.). St. Louis, MO: Mosby.

Redman, B. K. (2003). *Measurement tools in patient education* (2nd ed.). New York, NY: Springer.

Redman, B. K. (2004). *Advances in Patient Education.* New York: Springer.

Redman, B. K. (2006). *The practice of patient education: A case study approach* (10th ed.). St. Louis, MO: Mosby.

Redman, B. K. (2008). When is patient education unethical? *Nursing Ethics, 15*(6), 813–820.

Reiser, S. J. (1981). *Medicine and the reign of technology.* Cambridge, MA: Cambridge University Press.

Rice, E. G., & Okun, M. A. (1994). Older readers' processing of medical information that contradicts their beliefs. *Journal of Gerontology, 49*(3), 119–128.

Riddick, F. A., Jr. (2003). The code of medical ethics of the American Medical Association. *The Ochsner Journal, 5*(2), 6–10.

Roberts, K. (2004). Simplify, simplify: Tackling health literacy by addressing reading literacy. *American Journal of Nursing, 104*(3), 118–119.

Robinson, J. H., Callister, L. C., Berry, J. A., & Dearing, K. A. (2008). Patient-centered care and adherence: Definitions and applications to improve outcomes. *Journal of the American Academy of Nurse Practitioners, 20*(12), 600–607.

Roediger, H. L., & Karpicke, J. D. (2006). The power of testing memory: Basic research and implications for educational practice. *Perspectives on Psychological Science, 1*, 181–210.

Rogers, E. S., Wallace, L. S., & Weiss, B. D. (2006). Misperceptions of medical understanding in low-literacy patients: Implications for cancer prevention. *Cancer Control, 13*(3), 225–229.

Roland, J. (2008). Rationality and logic. *The Review of Metaphysics, 61*(3), 632–634.

Rolls, E. T., Horrak, J., Wade, D., & McGrath, J. (1994). Emotion-related learning in patients with social and emotional changes associated with frontal lobe damage. *Journal of Neurology, Neurosurgery and Psychiatry, 57*(12), 1518–1524.

Rosen, G. (1977). *Preventive medicine in the United States 1900–1975.* New York, NY: Prodist.

Rosenstock, I. M. (1966). Why people use health services. *Millbank Memorial Fund Quarterly, 44*(3), 94–127.

Rosenstock, I. M., Strecher, V. J., & Becker, M. H. (1988). Social learning theory and the health belief model. *Health Educator Quarterly, 15*(2), 175–183.

Ross, K. (2006). Psychology of learning and motivation: The advances in research and theory. *Psychology of Learning and Motivation, 46.*

Roter, D. L. (1977). Patient Participation in the patient-provider interaction: The effects of patient question asking on the quality of interaction, satisfaction and compliance. *Health Education and Behavior, 5*(4), 281–315.

Roter, D. L., Satashefsky-Margalit, R., & Rudd, R. (2001). Current perspectives on patient education in the US. *Patient Education and Counseling, 44*(1), 79–86.

Rudd, R. (2015). The evolving concept of health literacy: new direction for health literacy studies. *Journal of Communication in Healthcare, 8*(1), 7–9.

Rumelhart, D. E., & Ortony, A. (1977). The representation of knowledge in memory. In R. C. Anderson & R. J. Speiro (Eds.), *Schooling and the acquisition of knowledge.* Hillsdale, NJ: Erlbaum.

Rumsey, S., Hurford, D. P., & Cole, A. K. (2003). Influence of knowledge and religiousness on attitudes toward organ donation. *Transplant Proceedings, 35*(8), 2845–2850.

Sackett, D. L., Rosenberg, W. M., Gray, J. A., Haynes, R. B., & Richardson, W. S. (1996). Evidence-based medicine: What it is and what it isn't. *BMJ (Clinical Research Ed.), 312*(7023), 71–72.

Sandars, J., & Esmail, A. (2003). The frequency and nature of medical error in primary care: Understanding the diversity across studies. *Family Practice, 20*(3), 231–236.

Santrock, J. W. (2007). Cognitive development approaches. In E. Barrosse (Ed.), *A Topical Approach to Life-Span Development* (pp. 225–230). New York, NY: Beth Mejia.

Santrock, J. W. (2008). *A topical approach to life span development*. New York, NY: McGraw-Hill.

Saunders, W. (1992). The constructivist perspective: Implications and teaching strategies for science. *School Science and Mathematics, 92*, 136–141.

Save the Children. (2000). *State of the world's mothers (Save the Children)*. Westport, CT: Save the Children.

Schell, T. J. (1986). Cognitive conception of learning. *Review of Educational Research, 56*(4), 411–437.

Schillinger, D., Grumbach, K., Piette, J., et al. (2002). Association of health literacy with diabetes outcomes. *Journal of American Medical Association, 288*(4), 475–482.

Schwab, C. (2007). *The physician-patient relationship*. Available at: https://www.uthsc.edu/Medicine/legaledu/UT/factsheets/PhysicianPatientRelationship.pdf.

Schwartz, L. M., Woloshin, S., Black, W. C., & Welch, H. G. (1997). The role of numeracy in understanding the benefit of screening mammography. *Annuals of Internal Medicine, 127*(11), 966–972.

Schwartzberg, J. G. (2002). Low health literacy: What do your patients really understand? *Nursing Economics, 20*(3), 145–147.

Schwartzenberg, J. G. (2007). Communication techniques for patients with low health literacy: A survey of physicians, nurses, and pharmacists. *American Journal of Health Behavior, 31*(Suppl. 1), 96–104.

Schwartzenberg, J. G., Corrett, A., VanGeest, J., & Wolf, M. S. (2007). Communication techniques for patients with low health literacy: A survey of physicians, nurses, and pharmacists. *American Journal of Health Behavior, 31*(Suppl. 1), 96–104.

Schwartzenburg, J. G., VanGeest, J., & Wang, C., et al. (Eds.), (2005). *Understanding health literacy: Implications for medicine and public health (ed.)*. United States: AMA Press.

Secretary's Advisory Committee on National Health Promotion and Disease Prevention. (2009, November 3). *US Department of Health and Human Services*. Retrieved from Developing Healthy People 2020 on December 5, 2011 http://www.healthypeople.gov/hp2020/0bjectives/files/Draft20090bjectives.pdf.

Seligman, H. K., Wang, F. F., Palacios, J. L., et al. (2005). Physician notification of their diabetes patients' limited health literacy. *Journal of General Internal Medicine, 20*(11), 1001–1007.

Shanks, D. R. (2010). Learning from association to cognition. *Annual Review of Psychology, 61*(1), 273–301.

Shaw, S. J., Huebner, C., Armin, J., Orzech, K., & Vivian, J. (2009). The role of culture in health literacy and chronic disease screening and management. *Journal of Immigrant Minority Health, 11*, 460–467.

Shea, S. C. (2006). Is it really noncompliance? In S. C. Shea (Ed.), *Improving medication adherence: how to talk with patients about their medications* (pp. 33–48). Philadelphia, PA: Wolters Kluwer Health Inc.

Shiel, W.C. Jr., (n.d.) Medical definition of standard of care. Available at: https://www.medicinenet.com/script/main/art.asp?articlekey=33263.

Shuell, T. J. (1990). Phases of meaningful learning. *Review of Educational Research, 60*(4), 531–547.

Simonds, S. K. (1978). Health education: Facing issues of policy, ethics, and social justice. *Health Education Monographs*, 6(Suppl. 1), 18–27.

Simonton, D. K. (1985). Intelligence and personal influence in groups: Four nonlinear models. *Psychological Review*, 92(4), 532–547.

Simpson, M., Buckman, R., Stewart, M., Maguire, P., Lipkin, M., & Novack, D. (1991). Doctor-patient communication: The Toronto consensus statement. *British Medical Journal*, 303(6814), 1385–1387.

Skelton, A. M. (1997). Patient education for the millennium: Beyond and emancipation? *Patient Education and Counseling*, 31(2), 151–158.

Skevington, S. M., & Garro, L. (1995). *Psychology of Pain*. Oxford, England: John Wiley & Sons.

Skinner, B. F. (1966). Contingencies of reinforcement in the design of a culture. *Behavioral Science*, 11(3), 159–166.

Skinner, B. F. (1974). *About behaviorism*. New York, NY: Random House.

Skinner, B. F. (1991). *The behavior of organisms*. Acton, MA: Copley Publishing.

Slavin, R. E. (1995). A model of effective instruction. *Educational Forum*, 59(2), 166–176.

Smart, J. (2008). *Disability, Society, and the Individual* (2nd ed.). Austin, TX: Pro-Ed.

Smith, N. (2011). Patient Education: Determining a patient's readiness to learn. CINAHL Guide.

Smith, S. K., Dixon, A., Trevena, L., Nutbeam, D., & McCaffery, K. L. (2009). Exploring patient involvement in healthcare decision making across different education and functional health literacy groups. *Social Science and Medicine*, 69(12), 1805–1812.

Sorrell, J. M. (2006). Health literacy in older adults. *Journal of Psychosocial Nursing*, 44(3), 17–20.

Sousa, D. A. (2006). *How the Brain Learns*. Thousand Oaks, CA: Corwin Press.

Spann, S. (2016). The incredible costs of low health literacy.

Spath, P. L. (Ed.), (2008). *Engaging patients as safety partners: a guide for reducing errors and improving satisfaction*. Chicago, IL: Health Forum.

Speros, C. (2005). Health literacy: Concept analysis. *Journal of Advanced Nursing*, 50(6), 633–640.

Spiers, M. V., Kutzik, D. M., & Lamar, M. (2004). Variation in medication understanding among the elderly. *American Journal of Health-System Pharmacists*, 61(4), 373–380.

Spring, B. (2008). Health decision making: Lynchpin of evidence-based practice. *Medical Decision Making*, 28(6), 866–874.

Stableford, S., & Mettger, W. (2007). Plain language: A strategic response to the health literacy challenge. *Journal of Public Health Policy*, 28(1), 71–93.

Stewart, M. (2008). 5 Rights of Patient Education. In *A prescription for patient education: Assessing patient needs*. Joint Commission Resources Audio Conferences.

Stewart, M. (2009). *Becoming an expert in patient education*. IA: Baton Rouge.

Stewart, M., Meredith, L., Brown, J. B., & Galajda, J. (2000). The influence of older patient-physician communication on health and health-related outcomes. *Clinics on Geriatric Medicine*, 16(1), 25–36.

Stewart, M. N. (2008). Testing, testing 1,2,3-Patient education outcomes. In *A prescription for patient education: assessing patient needs*. Joint Commission Resources Audio Conferences.

Stewart, M. N. (2008). *5 rights of patient education*. Oklahoma City, OK: *Neural Perspectives Conference*.

Sthapornnanon, N., Sakulbumrungsil, R., Theeraroungchaisri, A., & Watcharadamrongkun, S. (2009). Social constructivist learning environment in an online professional practice course. *American Journal of Pharmaceutical Education*, *73*(1), 1–8.

Stone, M. A., Pound, E., Pancholi, A., Farooqi, A., & Khunti, K. (2005). Empowering patient with diabetes: A qualitative primary care study focusing on South Asians in Leicester, UK. *Family Practice*, *22*(6), 647–652.

Stonecypher, K. (2009). Creating a patient education tool. *The Journal of Continuing Education in Nursing*, *40*(10), 462–467.

Stuart-Hamilton, I. (2006). *The Psychology of Ageing: An Introduction*. London, U.K.: Jessica Kingsley Publishers. Retrieved from http://lib.myilibrary.com/Browse/open.asp?ID=92944&loc=102.

Sudore, R., & Schillinger, D. (2009). Interventions to improve care for patients with limited health literacy. *Journal of Clinical Management*, *16*(1), 20–29.

Sudore, R. L., Mehta, K. M., Simonsick, E. M., et al. (2006). Limited literacy in older people and disparities in health and healthcare access. *Journal of American Geriatrics Society*, *54*, 770–776.

Sullivan, M. (2003). The new subjective medicine: Taking the patient's point of view on health care and health. *Social Science and Medicine*, *56*(7), 1595–1604.

Swanson, L. (2007). New mental health services for deaf patients. *Canadian Medical Association Journal*, *176*(2), 160.

Syred, M. E. (1981). The abdication of the role of health education by hospital nurses. *Journal of Advanced Nursing*, *6*(1), 27–33.

Take steps now to reduce readmissions, ED visits within 30 days. (2009). Hospital. *Case Management*, *17*(5), 65–67.

Tang, P. C., & Lansky, D. (2005). The missing link: Bridging the patient-provider health information gap. *Health Affairs*, *24*(5), 1290–1295.

Tattersall, R. (1995). Patient education 2000: Take-home messages from this congress. *Patient Education and Counseling*, *26*(3), 373–377.

The Joint Commission. (2007). What did the doctor say? In *Improving health literacy to protect patient safety (The Joint Commission)*. Oakbrook Terrace, IL: Author.

Thompson, L. A., Knapp, C. A., Saliba, H., Guinta, N., Shenkman, E. A., & Nackashi, J. (2009). The impact of insurance on satisfaction and family-centered care for CSHCN. *Pediatrics*, *124*(Suppl 4), S407–S413.

Thorndike, E. (1932). *The fundamentals of learning*. New York, NY: Teachers College Press.

Thorndike, E. L. (1911). *Animal intelligence: experimental studies*. New York, NY: Macmillan.

Thorndike, E. L., Bregman, E. O., Tilton, J. W., & Wood, Y. E. (1928). *Adult learning*. New York, NY: Macmillan.

Tkacz, V. L., Metzgner, A., & Pruchnicki, M. C. (2008). Health literacy in pharmacy. *American Journal of Health System Pharmacist*, *65*(10), 974–981.

Tokarz, K. A. (2009). Patient education and self-advocacy: Queries and responses on pain management; erythromelalgia. *Journal of Pain and Palliative Care Pharmacotherapy, 23*(3), 295–297.

Tooth, L., Clark, M., & McKenna, K. (2000). Poor functional health literacy: The silent disability for older people. *Australasian Journal on Aging, 19*(1), 14–22.

Towle, A., & Godolphin, W. (1999). *Framework for teaching and learning informed shared decision making.* Retrieved from BMJ on December 30, 2011 from http://www.bmj.com/ content/319/7212/766. extract.

Trossman, S. (2010). Issues up close: Nurses promoting true health understanding through literacy. *American Nurse Today, 5*(9), 32–33.

Trostle, J. (1988). Medical compliance as an ideology. *Social Science and Medicine, 27*(12), 1299–1308.

Tuan, L. T. (2011). Matching and stretching learners' learning styles. *Journal Of Language Teaching & Research, 2*(2), 285–294.

Twanmoh, J. R., & Cunningham, G. P. (2006). When overcrowding paralyzes an emergency department. *Managed Care, 15*(6), 54–59.

US Department of Health and Human Services. (2008). *Health literacy improvement.* Retrieved from http://health.gov/communication/literacy/default.htm.

US Department of Health and Human Services. (1999). *Patient's bill of rights [Press release].* Retrieved from http://www.hhs.gov/news/press/1999pres/990412.html.

US Department of Health and Human Services National Institutes of Health Clinical Center, Patient bill of rights. Available at: https://clinicalcenter.nih.gov/participate/patientinfo/legal/bill_of_rights.html.

US Department of Labor. (2001). *Statistics about people with disabilities and employment.* Retrieved from http://www.dol.gov/odep/archives/ekOl/stats.htm.

U.S. Department of Health and Human Services, Office of Disease Prevention and Health Promotion (2010). National Action Plan to Improve Health Literacy. Washington, DC.

Untersmayr, E., & Jensen-Jarolim, E. (2006). The effect of gastric digestion on food allergy. *Current Opinion in Allergy and Clinical Immunology, 6*(3), 214–219.

Van de Borne, H. W. (1998). The patient from receiver of information to informed decision-maker! *Patient Education and Counseling, 34*(2), 89–102.

Veldtman, G. R., Matley, S. L., Kendall, L., Quirk, J., Gibbs, J. L., Parsons, J. M., et al. (2001). Illness understanding in children and adolescents with heart disease. *Western Journal of Medicine, 174*(3), 171–173.

Vernon, J. A., Trujillo, A., Rosenbaum, S., & DeBuono, B. (2007). *Low health literacy: implications for national health policy.* Washington, DC: George Washington University School of Public Health and Health Services.

Villaire, M., & Mayer, G. (2009). Health Literacy: The low-hanging fruit in health care reform. *Journal of Health Care Finance, 36*(2), 55–59.

Visser, A., Deccache, A., & Bensing, J. (2001). Patient education in Europe: United differences. *Patient Education and Counseling, 44*(1), 1–5.

Visser, A. P. (1996). Patient education and counseling: rights, duties, critics and credits. *Patient Education and Counseling, 28*(1), 1–3.

Wagner, E. (2004). *Part 1: The chronic care model [Video].* Available from http://www.researchchannel.org/prog/displayevent.aspx?rID=3877&flD=345.

Wagner, E. H., Austin, B. T., Davis, C., Hindmarsh, M., Schaefer, J., & Bonomi, A. (2001). Improving chronic illness care: Translating evidence into action. *Health Affairs, 20*(6), 64–78.

Waitzkin, H. (1984). Doctor-patient communication: Clinical implications of social scientific research. *Journal of the American Medical Association, 252*(17), 2441–2446.

Walford, S., & Alberti, K. G. (1985). Biochemical self-monitoring: promise, practice and problems. *Contemporary issues in clinical biochemistry, 2,* 200–213.

Watson, J. B. (1930). *Behaviorism* (Rev. ed.). New York, NY: WW Norton.

Watson, J. B., & Rayner, R. (1920). *Conditioned emotional reactions.* Retrieved from Classics in the History of Psychology http://psychclassics.yorku.ca/Watson/emotion.htm.

Webb, J., Davis, T. C., Bernadella, P., Clayman, M. L., Parker, R. M., Adler, D., et al. (2008). Patient-centered approach for improving prescription drug warning labels. *Patient Education and Counseling, 72*(3), 443–449.

Weekly, Physician's (2012). *Assessing medical decision-making capacity.* Available at: https://www.physiciansweekly.com/medical-decision-making-capacity.

Weiner, S. J., Barnet, B., Chang, T. L., & Daaleman, T. P. (2005). Processes for effective communication in primary care. *Annals of Internal Medicine, 142*(8), S709–S714.

Weinman, J., & Petrie', K.J., & Moss-Morris, R. (1996). The illness perception questionnaire: A new method for assessing the cognitive representation of illness. *Psychology and Health, 11,* 431–435.

Weinstein, N. D., Rutgers, U., & Cook, C. (1993). Testing four competing theories of health-protective behavior. *Health Psychology, 12*(4), 324–333.

Weiss, B. D. (2007). *Health Literacy and Patient Safety: Help patients understand* (2nd ed.). American Medical Association Foundation. Retrieved December 2, 2011 from http://www.ama-assn.org/amal/pub/upload/mm/367/healthlitclinicians.pdf.

Weiss, B. D., Blanchard, J. S., McGee, D. L., et al. (1994). Illiteracy among Medicaid recipients and its relationship to health care costs. *Journal of Health Care for the Poor and Underserved, 5*(2), 99–111.

White, J. (1999). Targets and systems of healthcare costs control. *Journal of Health Politics, Policy, and Law, 24*(4), 653–696.

White, S. (2008). *Assessing the nation's health literacy: Key concepts and findings of the national assessment of adult literacy.* (American Medical Association Foundation). Retrieved from AMA Foundation http://www.ama-assn.org/amal/pub/upload/mm/367 /hl_report_2008. pdf.

White, S., Chen, J., & Atchison, R. (2008). Relationship of preventative health practices and health literacy: A national study. *American Journal of Health Behavior, 32*(3), 227–242.

Whitehead, D. (2006). Health Promotion in the practice setting: Findings from a review of clinical issues. *Worldviews on Evidence-based Nursing, 3*(4), 165–184.

Williams, A., Lindsell, C., Rue, L., & Blomkalns, A. (2007). Emergency department education improves patient knowledge of coronary artery disease risk. *Preventive Medicine, 44*(6), 520–525.

Willshaw, D. J., & Buckingham, J. T. (1990). An assessment of Marr's theory of the as a temporary memory store. *Philosophical Transactions: Biological Sciences,* *329*(1253), 205–215.

Wingate, S. (1990). Patient perceptions of their learning needs. *Dimensions of Critical Care Nursing, 9*(2), 112–118.

Wisconsin Public Health. (2002). *Containing Wisconsin public health costs (Wisconsin Public Health & Health Policy Institute Brief).* Wisconsin: Wisconsin Public Health.

Wlodkowski, R. J. (2008). *Enhancing adult motivation to learn: a comprehensive guide for teaching all adults.* San Francisco, CA: John Wiley and Sons.

Wolf, M. S., Davis, T. C., Shrank, W., et al. (2007). To err is human: Patient misinterpretations of prescription drug label instruction. *Patient Education and Counseling, 67*(3), 293–300.

Yancey, A., Tanjasini, S., Klein, M., & Tunder, J. (1995). Increased cancer screening behavior in women of color by culturally sensitive video exposure. *Preventive Medicine, 24*(2), 142–148.

Zins, J. E., Weissberg, P. P., Wang, M. E., & Walberg, H. J. (Eds.), (2004). *Building Academic Success on Social and Emotional Learning: What Does the Research Say?.* New York: Teachers College Press.

Zull, J. E. (2006). Key aspects of how the brain learns. In S. Johnson & J. Taylor (Eds.), *The neuroscience of adult learning: new directions for adult and continuing education* (110th ed., pp. 3–10). San Francisco, CA: Jossey Bass.

Note: Page numbers followed by *f* indicate figures, *t* indicate tables, and *b* indicate boxes.